Shredded Beast

Get lean. Build muscle. Be a man.

David De Las Morenas

ISBN-13: 978-1496037084

ISBN-10: 1496037081

Waiver of Liability

You have purchased or obtained *Shredded Beast* ("The Guide" or "Guide"), written by David De Las Morenas ("DLM"). In so doing, you acknowledge and agree to the terms and conditions set forth below.

1. PHYSICAL ACTIVITY READINESS. You, represent that: (a) You are voluntarily engaging in physical exercise, are in good physical condition and have no disabilities, diseases, illnesses or other conditions that could prevent You from exercising and using DLM's Guide without injuring yourself/themselves or impairing Your health; (b) You have consulted a licensed physician concerning an exercise program that will not expose You to risk of injury or impairment to Your health; and (c) Your physician has approved your contemplated activities. You acknowledge that DLM has not given You any medical advice and You are relying solely on the advice of Your licensed physicians regarding the ability to use the DLM's Guide. You agree to consult with Your physician prior to making any dietary changes or use of any food supplements.

2. ACKNOWLEDGEMENT OF RISK. You represent that You understand that engaging in physical exercise and the carrying out DLM's Guide includes an inherent risk of minor or major life threatening injury to persons and property, and death.

You also understand that risk of injury to persons and property includes, but is not limited to, injuries arising from or relating to (a) the use or carrying out by You of DLM's Guide including but not limited to while using exercise equipment and machines and other formal or informal health club facilities or Your home, home fitness or workout room, health club, gym; (b) participation by You in any supervised and unsupervised activities, programs, classes, events other than those included in DLM's Guide; (c) any personal training, instruction, supervision or dietary recommendations by DLM; (d) medical disorders that may occur from use of DLM's Guide such as heart attack, stroke, death, heat stress, sprains, strains, broken bones, and torn muscles, tendons and ligaments among others; (e) accidents that may occur anywhere in or around any premises (including but not limited to Your home, home fitness or workout room, health club, gym, exercise areas) while carrying out DLM's Guide and (f) theft or loss of property while carrying out DLM's Guide. Accidental injuries include those caused by You or by other persons and those, for example, of a slip and fall nature. You agree to use due care when carrying out DLM's Guide.

3. INDEMNIFICATION AND HOLD HARMLESS. You agree to defend, indemnify and hold DLM harmless from any causes of action relating to this Agreement for DLM's Guide, including but not limited to all lawsuits, claims and legal action.

About the Author

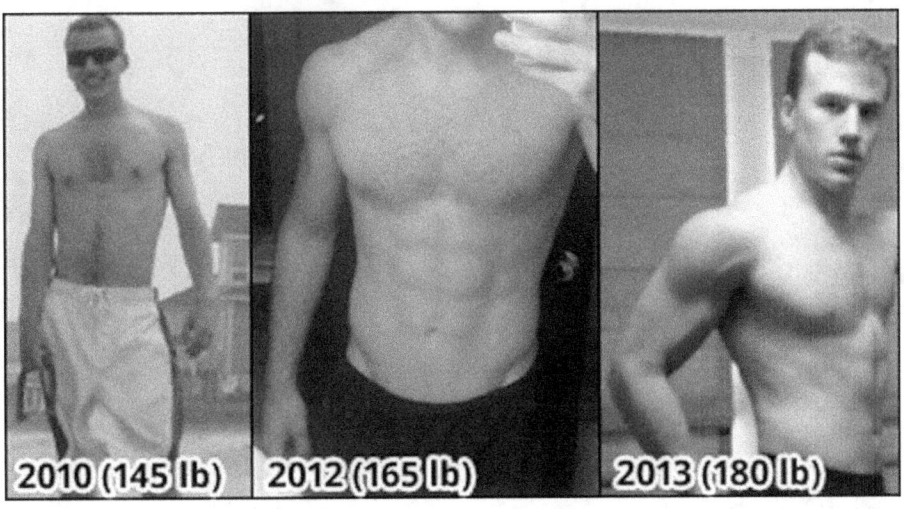

2010 (145 lb) 2012 (165 lb) 2013 (180 lb)

Hi, I'm David.

I trained for various sports throughout my childhood, but didn't begin lifting weights until I was about 18. I didn't see any results, though.

A few years later, while living abroad in Madrid, I befriended a bodybuilder. Since then I've been obsessed with lifting weights and studying the sciences of muscle growth and fat loss. This obsession led me to transforming my body from a skinny and weak 145 pounds to a lean, muscular, and strong 180 pounds.

This transformation radically enhanced my confidence and outlook on life. I quit my job as a Software Solutions Engineer to help others experience the same transformation. So far I've successfully helped thousands of men through my work as a personal trainer, my website (**www.HowToBeast.com**), and my books on men's fitness and self-improvement.

Buyer Bonus

Thank you for buying *Shredded Beast.* Visit **www.HowToBeast.com/50-Reasons-Youre-Still-Skinny** to download *50 Reasons You're Still Skinny* for free. This eBook contains a comprehensive list of the most common muscle building mistakes men make.

Contents

Introduction

Why Building a Superior Body is an Essential Part of Being a Man

Let's be honest: most men get into fitness because they want to look good naked.

I didn't care about lowering my cholesterol levels or reducing the risk of chronic disease when I started lifting weights. Yes, those are actual benefits of training. But I was in college, and I wanted to look good so I could get laid more.

I'm betting your story isn't too different. In fact, it's probably exactly the same. I think it's the number one reason dudes get into weight lifting. The exception would be old guys with back pain. If you're a 65 year old guy with back pain, chances are this book isn't for you. Do yourself a favor and put it down.

But attracting more, hotter women is the best reason for sculpting a ripped, jacked body, right?

Looking back now, after having transformed my body, the answer is a loud, resounding no.

The real value in improving your physique isn't even physical. It has nothing to do with your body. The reason is that it teaches you how to set goals and persist until they're accomplished. It ingrains the habit of setting and achieving goals into your conscious.

The value of this habit cannot be overstated. Overcoming constant resistance and plowing through obstacles in order to arrive at a particular outcome is an essential part of being a man. You'll need to follow this same process in order to land any great job, start your own company, or produce any new object of value. Nothing worthwhile comes easy.

Building your body is no different. You must first choose exactly what you want. For most guys this is similar: larger-than-average muscles with clearly visible definition. And then you must get there. That's the hard part. That's why most guys look like shit. If it were easy then we'd all be walking around with bodies of Greek gods.

However, I think you'll find the approach I offer in this book effective. Its effectiveness is a direct result of the addictive nature of my weight lifting habit. I've figured out how I got myself addicted to lifting weights and eating a diet conducive to muscle growth and fat loss. It's the same method I've successfully implemented for many of my personal training clients.

Keep reading and I'll show you how it's done. But first, I leave you with a great quote from the greatest of all time:

The resistance that you fight physically in the gym and the resistance that you fight in life can only build a strong character.

- Arnold Schwarzenegger

Chapter 1

The Top 3 Fat Loss Mistakes Guys Make

At least 95% of guys at your gym aren't making any progress. They're just spinning their wheels.

They get to the gym, run on the treadmill for a bit, hit the bench press, and grind out a few curls before calling it a day. They might follow a routine. They might even go through periods of *watching their diet* (whatever that means) or buying supplements that are supposed to *burn fat* and *build muscle fast*!

But it's all bullshit, complete and utter bullshit. And you know it. Be honest: how much have you improved your body over the last six months? The last year? The last two years?

Maybe you've done a bit, but if you're reading this book then you aren't completely satisfied with your progress. I know that much.

The problem is that almost everyone is taking shots in the dark. They're combining something their friend told them with something they read on the internet. And then they're adding in a tip or two from the personal trainer or buff bro at the local gym.

They combine all of these things and end up with a big mish-mash of garbage, when what they really need is a simple approach that they can put into place and forgot about. Yes, exercise science is progressing, but not at an astronomical rate.

I promise you'd be better off if you picked a single basic, fundamental approach and then followed it for the next year. During that year, you must ignore every tip or article that's shared with you on Facebook, emailed to you by a friend, or offered to you at the gym.

I'm not saying that I'm right and everyone else is wrong, just that when you combine random particles of different methods you're likely to tweak something that already works before giving it a chance.

In this book I offer a simple approach that's backed by science and easy to follow. Not just easy, but addictive. You'll want to keep going. And that fact alone is what will guarantee you the results you desire.

So while program hopping, excessive dietary tweaking, and all-around fitness ADD might be the single biggest mistake guys make, I want to share some more specific mistakes I see all the time. I'll start with the three most common fat loss mistakes.

1. Going too heavy on the cardio

It's an undeniable fact that cardio has become synonymous with weight loss for most people.

And while cardio does have various health benefits, magical weight loss is definitely not one of them. Going hard for 30 minutes to an hour on the elliptical, bike, or treadmill every day of the week isn't going to melt fat away. But it *is* going to burn you out mentally.

Furthermore, the metabolic benefits of cardio are minimal. This means that the amount of calories you burn over the course of the day (while not doing cardio) isn't going to increase much, if at all, from increased cardio (1).

So that leaves the actual calories you burn during a session of cardio as the main reason for doing it to lose weight. And let's be completely honest: it's WAY easier to not eat a Snickers bar, a bag of chips, or a couple slices of bread (all about 300 calories) than it is to run on the treadmill for 30 minutes (to burn about 300 calories).

My point is that dietary restriction is far more effective than cardio in regards to weight loss.

2. Not lifting heavy weights

I can't even count the number of times a buddy of mine stopped lifting weights or chose to lift only light weights because he wanted to lose fat.

I think it's because we associate heavy weights with building muscle. When you decide your goal is to cut weight (and not gain muscle), you naturally assume that you need to stop lifting heavy.

First of all, that's terrible logic. Second of all, foregoing lifting heavy weights while losing body weight will result in your body shedding muscle along with the fat (2).

This is because your body doesn't have a reason to hold onto the muscle. You aren't activating a maximal number of muscle fibers or motor units if you aren't lifting heavy. This means that your body will have no reason to maintain your muscle mass, and begin to shed it along with the fat.

It takes a lot of time and energy to build muscle. The last thing you want to do is give up your hard earned muscle during a period of weight loss. Not only will you be weaker afterwards, but you'll look like shit. An aesthetically pleasing body combines ample muscle mass with a low body fat percentage (i.e. you have muscle and there's only a small layer of fat covering it).

When you take away the muscle along with the fat, you begin to approach skinny fat (a heinous condition marked by small amounts of both muscle and fat – skinny, but without definition). Trust me: you don't want to be skinny fat.

3. Obsessing over the scale

I get it. You have some extra belly fat that you want to get rid of. Who doesn't?

But you must be careful. If you get obsessed with seeing weight drop off the scale you run a high risk of unhealthy weight loss.

Starving yourself and going heavy on the cardio is definitely an effective way to drop weight fast. But remember, dropping weight shouldn't be the goal – cutting fat should be.

You must combine the almighty scale with the mirror and the weights. What I mean is that if your weight on the scale is dropping, you're seeing more muscle definition in the mirror, and you're not getting weaker in the gym, then chances are you're cutting fat and maintaining muscle. This is the goal – keep it at the forefront of your mind.

Chapter 2

The Top 3 Muscle Building Mistakes Guys Make

Now let's flip the script and examine the other side of the coin: building muscle.

While fat loss is undeniably the top goal for men and women today, I'm hoping building muscle will make a comeback for men.

It's time to get over the desire to look like Justin Bieber or any other skinny teenage pop star. Sure, women think he's cute. But they want to squeeze him and cuddle with him, not have sex. For that, they want a manly man.

Having muscle mass and the brute strength that comes along with it is both practical and masculine, not to mention healthy. Furthermore, it doesn't matter how skinny you are – if you don't have a solid base of muscle then you won't look good naked (do I have to explain the evils of skinny fat again?).

Without further ado, here are the top three most common muscle building mistakes guys make.

1. Overloading on protein shakes

Protein has become synonymous with muscle.

And while protein does contain the amino acids that act as the building blocks for muscle, it's essential to recognize how much of it you actually need to consume daily in order to maximize your muscle building potential.

Bodybuilding recommendations are bogus. Eating one gram of protein per pound of bodyweight or more each day is excessive.

While it's not going to hurt you physically, it *is* going to hurt you financially, because protein sources are far more expensive than fats or carbohydrates.

The current scientific recommendation for maximum daily protein intake for strength athletes is about 0.8 grams per pound (1.75 g/kg) of bodyweight (3). I believe this number is even a bit high. But it's a good number to shoot for to ensure you're providing your body what it needs to build muscle optimally.

The important thing to realize is that you can achieve this number by incorporating a source of protein (chicken, meat, fish, eggs, etc.) into each of your meals. You don't need to rely on protein shakes.

2. Lifting weights 5 or 6 days per week

We all know that lifting weights leads to the body's anabolic response that results in hypertrophy (the synthesis of new muscle tissue).

I'm not debating this point. But using backwards logic, people often use this as justification for lifting weights almost every single day.

More lifting = more muscle gains, right?

Wrong. The anabolic period takes place over roughly a 36 hour period after you lift (4). By slamming more and more lifting sessions into this window you aren't doing yourself any favors.

The anabolic processes in our bodies require proper rest and nutrition to work at maximum capacity, not lifting more weights. The take home lesson here is: go hard in the gym, and then focus on resting and eating to recover and build muscle. This way you can go just as hard during your next session, if not even harder.

3. Doing too many different exercises (aka confusing your muscles)

Muscle confusion is a concept that's gained popularity in recent years.

It revolves around the concept that by constantly switching the exercises you're doing, your muscles won't be able to get used to them, and then they'll keep growing as a result.

It's complete and utter bullshit.

Muscles don't have brains in them. You aren't confusing anyone, except maybe yourself.

What we do know, however, is that by focusing on getting stronger across a small set of exercises, you *will* build muscle efficiently. To understand this it's important to note the two main ways you get stronger for any given exercise.

The first way is via neural adaptations. When you do a new exercise for the first 10-20 times, you'll always see rapid increases in strength. Don't be fooled, this isn't because your body synthesizes massive amount of muscle tissue when it encounters a new exercise. This is happening because your brain and nervous system are familiarizing themselves with the movement, and getting more efficient at doing it, with roughly the same amount of muscle (5).

The second way your body adapts and becomes stronger at a particular exercise is via hypertrophy – by building new muscle tissue (5).

So when you constantly switch between exercises, you'll acquire the neural efficiency for a wide range of exercises but neglect most of the muscle hypertrophy that you could achieve if you just stuck with a handful of movements that hit every muscle in your body.

Chapter 3

Why *Shredded Beast* is the Solution to these Mistakes

Shredded Beast is the culmination of all of my weight training and dieting experiences: my own transformation and the transformations of my friends, family members, and personal training clients.

The main reasons most guys fail on their quests to building a better body are clear to me. I covered six of them on the previous pages. But, in reality, almost every mistake can be categorized into three areas: training, nutrition, and motivation.

Shredded Beast answers all three of these (in addition to the 6 aforementioned mistakes). It offers easy to follow, flexible nutrition concepts, an addictive approach to weight lifting, and a framework that will get you motivated from the start. It works because it gets you quick results, and then offers a sustainable approach to gradually improving your physique at a consistent rate over the long haul.

The initial results serve to get you hooked and pumped to continue. This is what I call *Phase 1: The Shred*. During this phase you'll quickly cut fat until you reach an acceptable level of leanness. You're creating the base for your masterpiece – a blank canvas, if you will.

After this period, you'll enter *Phase 2: The Beast*. At this point, your strength training becomes the focus. Now that you're at an acceptable level of body fat, you can shift all of your focus to getting stronger and mastering a set of beastly exercises. You'll remove the dietary restrictions you followed during Phase 1 and embrace your new lifestyle, where eating a lot of food is not just okay, but encouraged.

Because you're starting at a healthy body fat level and getting stronger, any weight gain that occurs during Phase 2 will be in the form of added muscle, not fat.

Are you ready to go?

Good, let's get it.

Next I'll cover the principles that will serve as your foundation before getting into the nitty-gritty of the program itself.

Chapter 4

The Only Way to Guarantee Fat Loss and Muscle Growth: Nutrition

If there's one simple fitness concept I wish everyone would get through their thick skulls, it's definitely the following:

The calorie is king.

Let me explain. There are three simple rules that solve the mystery of changes in bodyweight (6).

1. If you consume more calories than you expend, weight is gained.

2. If you consume fewer calories than you expend, weight is lost.

3. If you consume the same number of calories as you expend, weight is maintained.

And there you have it – nutrition's greatest mystery is solved with simple math. In the contradictory world of fitness where anything goes, this is one rule you can always count on. If people understood this they would never ask:

What's the best food to lose weight?

What foods should I avoid?

Will eating at night cause weight gain?

Are smaller, frequent meals better for losing weight?

...or any other weight related questions you can think of

But people are stupid and don't like thinking for themselves. They want other people to guide them and give them the answers. And that's the reason all of these supplement companies and nutrition experts can make money. They thrive off the ignorance of the general population.

If you just keep this one simple concept in the back of your head, you'll avoid constant fitness-induced headaches and start to make better dietary choices instantly.

The Lazy Man's Approach to Gaining and Losing Weight

Before I get into calculating how many calories you should eat to lose weight and cut fat or gain weight and build muscle, I want to offer an alternative – for the lazy men.

But first realize that having a caloric goal and keeping a rough count of your calories is ideal. It's the only way to guarantee the outcome you desire. And it's really easy (I'll offer my approach below). But if the mere thought of tracking calories makes you sick to your stomach, then follow this advice.

To lose weight (and cut fat):

- Eat three meals per day (don't snack)

- Focus the meals around protein, with only small amounts of carbs and fats

- Stop eating when you're full (not stuffed, just satisfied)

To gain weight (and build muscle):

- Eat four meals per day

- Incorporate a lot of proteins, carbs, and fats into each meal

- Eat until your full (stuffed is okay if you're having trouble gaining weight)

I'll add the additional advice that tracking your calories (as I describe below) for a month or so to get an idea of how much you should be eating, and then switching to *The Lazy Man's Approach* afterwards is much more effective than going lazy from the start.

So how many calories should I eat?

How much you should eat depends on whether you're trying to gain, lose, or maintain your weight.

Regardless, you must first calculate your RMR (Resting Metabolic Rate – the number of calories your body expends in a completely sedentary state). A simple formula to calculate this number is:

RMR = Bodyweight (in pounds) x 10

Or for the metrically aware: RMR = Bodyweight (in kg) x 22

Example: RMR = 175 lb. x 10 = 1750 calories

Next, select the appropriate activity level multiplier from the table below.

Multiplier	Activity Level
1.2 - 1.3	Very Light (Light daily activity and no exercise)
1.5 - 1.6	Low Active (Light daily activity and exercise 1-3 days/week)
1.6 - 1.7	Active (Moderate daily activity and exercise 3-5 days/week)
1.9 - 2.1	High Active (Intense daily activity and exercise 6-7 days/week)

Once you know your RMR and activity level multiplier you can easily calculate your TDEE (Total Daily Energy Expenditure).

TDEE = RMR x Activity Level

Example: Active (RMR taken from the above example), TDEE = 1750 x 1.6 = 2800 calories

This is approximately the number of calories you expend each day (15). The final step is to adjust this number to be in line with your goal:

Goal	How Much to Eat Each Day
Build Muscle	TDEE x 1.1 (10% surplus)
Lose Fat	TDEE x 0.8 (20% deficit)

Example: Weight gain (TDEE taken from the above example), 2800 x 1.1 = 3080 calories

I recommend a 20% deficit for losing and only a 10% surplus for gaining because, the body cannot realistically add more than half a pound of muscle per week, while higher rates of healthy weight loss are possible (16).

To ensure that the number you've calculated is accurate you should weigh yourself every two weeks, under the same conditions. Generally this means after waking up and using the bathroom, but before eating or drinking anything. Any more frequently will only cause confusion. Fluctuations in water weight, among other factors, affect your bodyweight on a day-to-day basis (17).

Depending on your change in weight, adjust your calories. If you're trying to build muscle but not gaining any weight: add 200 calories. If you're trying to cut fat but not losing weight: subtract 200 calories. It's important to keep the adjustments small (200 calories) because over-adjustment can lead to:

1. Fat gain: As much as you want to pack on 20 pounds of muscle each week, anything above about half a pound will be purely fat.

2. Muscle loss: If you want to cut fat, the same principle applies.

Losing over two pounds per week will lead to shedding hard-earned muscle along with the fat.

How do I track my calories?

Understanding the principle is one thing. Actually applying it is a whole different ball game.

And there's only one way: you must count your calories. Before you get flustered, give up, and return this book – I'll show you an easy way to estimate the number of calories you eat every day. No weighing your foods or any bullshit like that, I promise. You only need a rough estimate.

Just follow these 2 steps:

1. Download an app on your smartphone. I use *Calorie Counter* by *FatSecret*. They have a website you can use if you don't have a smartphone (**www.fatsecret.com**).

2. After each meal, enter the foods you ate into the app.

That's all. However, being able to estimate the quantity of your foods will prove useful (when you enter a food you ate into the app, it's going to ask you how much you ate). Refer to the following three rules:

1. A cup is about the size of your clenched fist. This is commonly used to measure liquids, rice, noodles, and other carbs.

2. A tablespoon is about the size of a golf ball. This is commonly used to measure butter, olive oil, peanut butter, and other fats.

3. Three ounces is about the size of a deck of cards. This is commonly used to measure meat, fish, chicken, and other proteins.

There you have it. I'll cover how to apply this to the *Shredded Beast* protocol once we get to the program itself.

Chapter 5

The Only Way to Guarantee Fat Loss and Muscle Growth: Training

The same way I boiled nutrition down to a single sentence, I can do the same for training:

The only thing that matters is getting stronger.

There are millions of different variables in play when it comes to weight lifting: exercise selection, rep range, sets, repetition tempo, volume, etc. – the list goes on and on. But rather than weighing yourself down and getting caught up in all the bullshit, if you focus solely on getting stronger, you'll be well on your way to a lean, muscular body.

Here are the three reasons why:

1. Getting stronger while losing weight = cutting fat, not muscle

I already covered this in the fat loss mistakes chapter, but I'll reiterate what I said.

If you lose weight but don't focus on gaining, or at least maintaining strength, you're at a high risk that the weight loss will be a combination of fat and muscle. This is bad. You want weight loss to be 100% fat, or as close to that as possible.

Lifting weights provides the stimulus your body needs to maintain high rates of muscle protein synthesis, and not shed muscle along with the fat.

2. Getting stronger while gaining weight = gaining muscle, not fat

This is the other side of the coin. If you gain weight, but don't get any stronger, your weight gain will be mainly fat.

The same way you need to give your body a reason to hold onto muscle mass when cutting weight, you need to give it a reason to synthesize new muscle tissue when gaining weight.

When you're gaining weight, by definition, you're in a caloric surplus – your body has more energy than it needs to perform its regular daily functions. You must ensure that this extra energy is put towards building muscle. The only way to do this is to use the extra energy as fuel to lift heavier weights at the iron temple.

3. It turns working out into an addictive game and ensures consistency

Last, but not least, when you focus on lifting more weight than you did last time you were at the gym, you turn strength training into a game.

Every time you step onto the gym floor you're competing against your previous best. And we men are competitive creatures. We thrive on improvement and a desire to win. With weight lifting you win by adding another 5 or 10 pounds to the bar.

Seeing visual changes in your body is powerful, and it's the reason we all got started, but it's not enough to keep us motivated for years of lifting weights and eating well. While keeping a goal physique in the back of your head is good, you must use your daily, weekly, and monthly increases in strength as the motivation you need to keep pushing on.

You can measure these increases in strength far better than you can measure the gradual changes in the mirror. Use this to your advantage, because changes in strength are ultimately what will lead to the beastly arms, coconut shoulders, thick back, rounded chest, and six pack abs you're working your ass off for.

Chapter 6

The Only 5 Exercises a Man Needs

Clearly getting stronger should be the aim of every man's exercise. And with only that knowledge most men would be making far better progress than they are today. But by adding in one additional caveat – success is guaranteed.

Recall from the chapter about muscle building mistakes that doing too many different exercises won't achieve anything besides stunting your muscle growth, because you're effectively trading gains in muscle mass for gains in neural efficiency.

This fact begs a question to be asked: if I should focus on only a handful of exercises, which ones are best? The answer is the following five movements.

These movements combine to hit every muscle in your body. And they won't only lead to an aesthetically pleasing and balanced physique, but they'll also drastically improve your athletic performance and functional strength in the process. They each represent one of the five fundamental human motions.

For each motion, I've included a preferred exercise, the muscles it targets, a detailed description of how to execute that exercise, and a list of alternatives. Needless to say, these movements will form the bulk of your *Shredded Beast* program.

1. The Squat

Preferred Exercise: Barbell Box Squat

Primary Muscles Worked: Quadriceps, Hamstrings, Glutes

Why:

The squat is widely accepted as the most essential exercise any man can do.

It's also commonly misrepresented as a lower body movement. In reality, it requires the concerted effort of every muscle in your body, save the chest and arms, to execute properly.

If you play a sport, you'll derive far more performance improvements from the squat than any other exercise. If you want to look good naked, it's still the most important, because it builds a solid muscular base that every other exercise will depend upon.

Moreover, to execute a squat properly you must address common muscle imbalances – the primary source of poor posture in men today. So your posture will improve as well.

I chose the barbell box squat as the preferred exercise for two main reasons (vs. a regular squat without a box):

1. Proper form is much simpler (you'll always get low enough and your heels will never leave the ground, among other things).

2. It builds explosive power, because you start from a dead stop at the bottom of each rep.

If you're not convinced, consider the fact that every member of the famed *Westside Barbell* powerlifting team uses the box squat year-round. They only squat without a box at their actual competitions.

How:

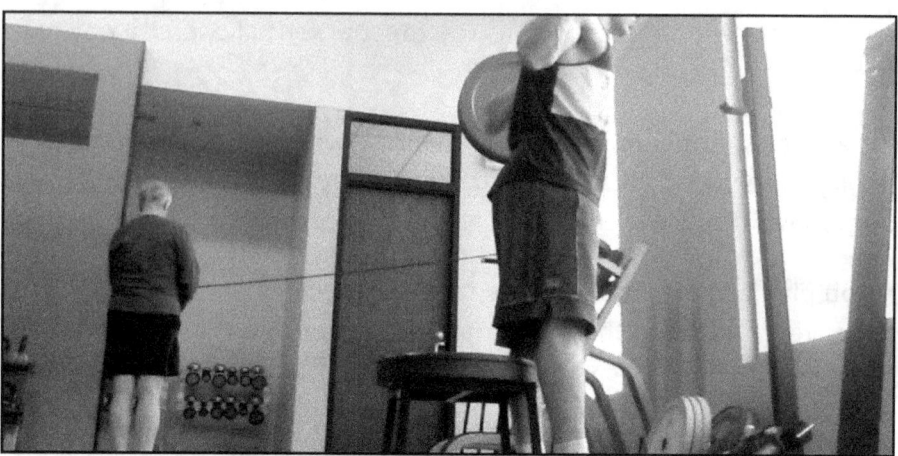

1. Position a box a few steps behind the squat rack. The "box" can really be anything, but it must be capable of supporting a lot of weight and be at a height so that your hips are level with (or just below) your knees when you're seated. As you can see, I use a short box with a 45 lb. weight on top of it.

2. Grab the barbell with an overhand grip just wider than shoulder width, move your body underneath it, and place it on your upper back.

2. Lift it from the rack with a firm grip (keeping your shoulder blades and elbows pulled back).

3. Take a few steps back, position your feet just wider than shoulder width apart, point your slightly outwards, and your heels within an inch of the box.

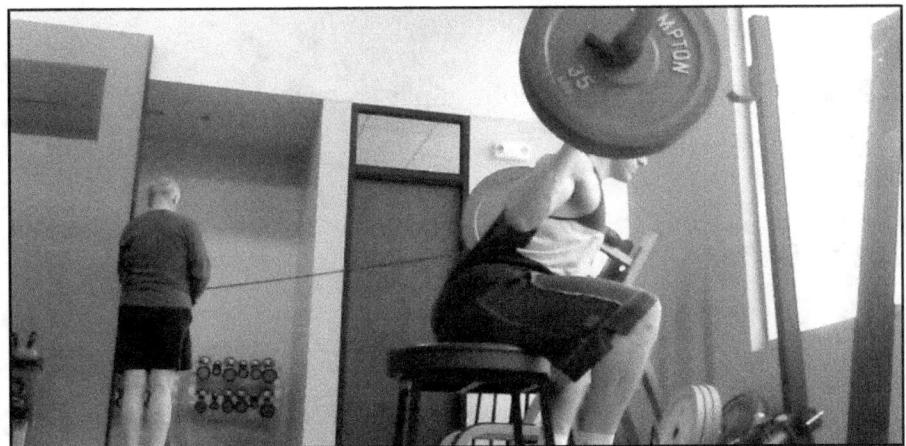

4. Inhale, tighten your abdomen and fill it with air, and sit back onto the box (keeping your feet flat, abs tight, and chest up).

5. Pause on the box for a split second, keeping your entire body tight.

6. Exhale and push through your heels to stand up.

Common Mistakes:

1. Heels coming off the floor at the bottom of the movement (your entire foot must remain in contact with the floor throughout the whole movement).

2. Sitting down instead of back (your butt and hips should move backwards as you lower your body). Think about how you sit on the toilet – that tends to be correct form.

3. Bouncing off the box (sit down slowly, rest for a split second, and then explode up – bouncing can damage your spine).

Alternatives:

1. Barbell Squat (no box)

2. Barbell Front Squat

3. Barbell Lunge (or Dumbbell Lunge)

4. Barbell Split Squat (or Dumbbell Split Squat)

5. Dumbbell Goblet Squat

2. The Deadlift

Preferred Exercise: Romanian Deadlift

Primary Muscles Worked: Hamstrings, Glutes, Upper Back

Why:

The deadlift mimics picking something heavy off of the floor. It will build your back, butt, and hamstrings. These are commonly weak areas in men that lead to slouching and poor posture.

Also, studies have shown the butt is often the first body part women notice on a man. Squats and deadlifts will combine to give you a booty that brings all the girls to the yard.

I've chosen the Romanian Deadlift (as opposed to the traditional deadlift), because I find it easier to teach (especially in written form). It's still tremendously effective.

How:

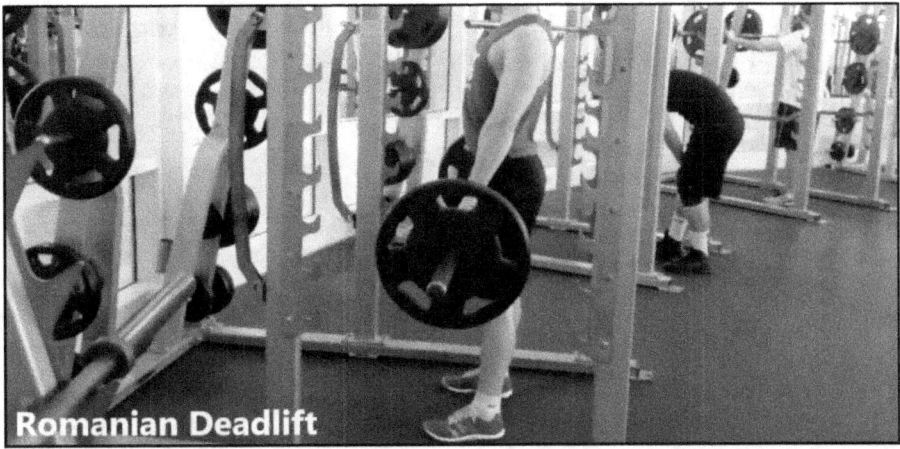

Romanian Deadlift

1. Grab the barbell with an overhand grip just wider than shoulder width, lift it from the rack, and take a couple of steps back.

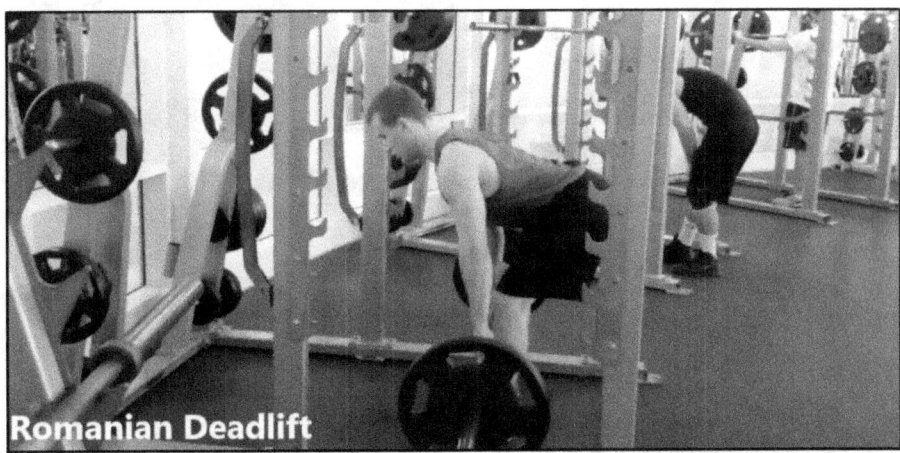

Romanian Deadlift

2. Keeping your abs tight and sucked in, your shoulder blades pinched back, and a slight bend in your knees – inhale and allow the weight to drop down while sticking your butt back.

3. When you feel a strong stretch in your hamstrings – exhale, stand up, and squeeze your butt forward to return to the starting position.

Common Mistakes:

1. Allowing the bar to come forward off of your legs (it should remain in contact with, and slide down, the front of your legs throughout the entire motion).

2. Rounding your back (your back should be straight throughout, focus on keeping your chest proud and facing up and your abs tight to prevent this).

Alternatives:

1. Traditional Barbell Deadlift

2. Trap Bar Deadlift

3. Dumbbell Deadlift

3. The Overhead Press

Preferred Exercise: Standing Barbell Shoulder Press

Primary Muscles Worked: Shoulders, Triceps, Upper Chest

Why:

The standing shoulder press will develop your shoulders, triceps, and upper chest. Also, because you're standing, your gluteal and abdominal muscles are needed to stabilize the body, resulting in a stronger core. It's also my favorite exercise.

How:

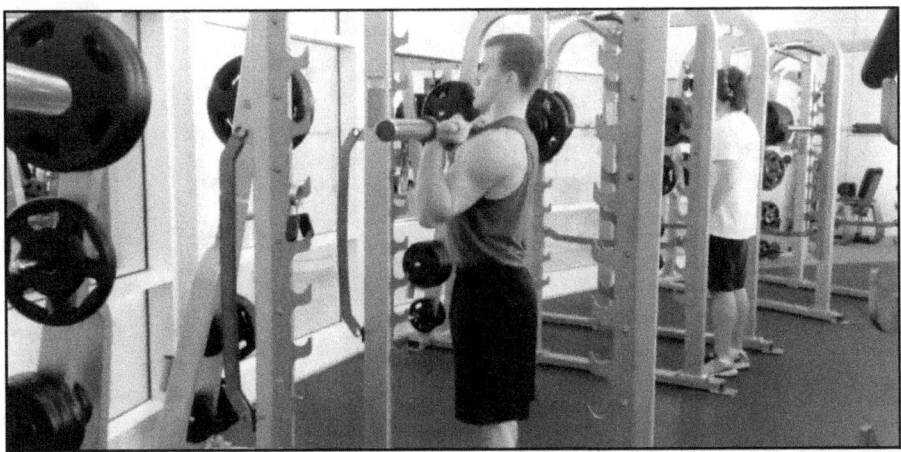

1. Grab the barbell with an overhand grip just wider than shoulder width, lift it from the rack.

2. Rest it on your upper chest with your elbows pointing a bit forward and a slight backward bend in your wrists.

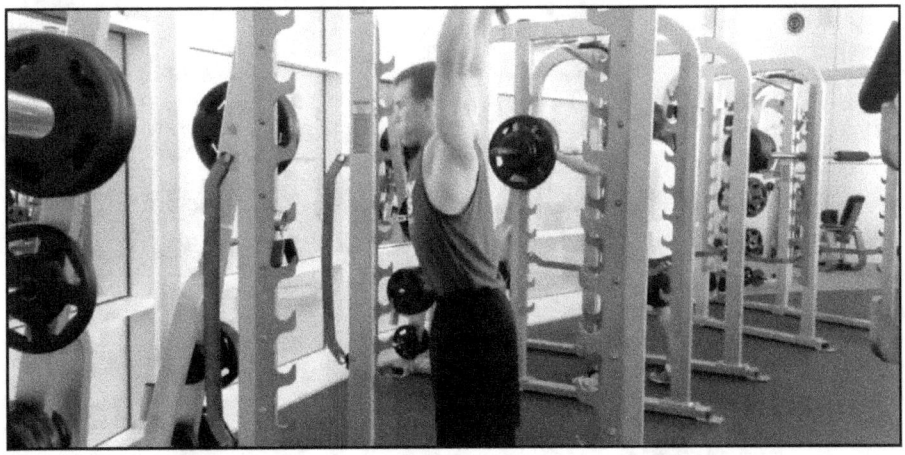

3. Exhale and press the bar upwards, moving your head and body underneath it as you go – so that when your elbows lock out, the bar is directly overhead.

4. Inhale and lower the bar back down to your upper chest.

Common Mistakes:

1. Allowing your back to round (keep your abs tight and your butt contracted to create a stable base and avoid this mistake).

2. Not pressing the bar directly and vertically overhead (make sure the bar ends directly overhead, not out in front of you).

Alternatives:

1. Seated Barbell Shoulder Press

2. Standing Dumbbell Shoulder Press

3. Seated Dumbbell Shoulder Press

4. The Chest Press

Preferred Exercise: Barbell Bench Press

Primary Muscles Worked: Chest, Triceps, Front Shoulders

Why:

Let's be honest, who isn't bench pressing already?

If you're completely unaware, it's the best exercise for adding mass and strength to your chest. It also crushes the triceps and front of the shoulders.

How:

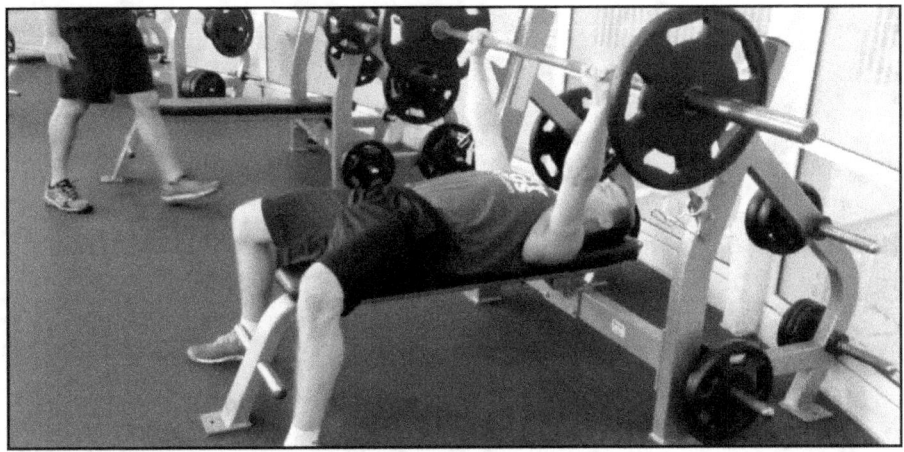

1. Lying flat on a bench with your feet flat on the floor, grab the bar firmly outside of shoulder width.

2. Pull your shoulder blades back so that they create a stable base to press from (your spine shouldn't be in contact with the bench, just your ass and shoulder blades).

3. Lift it from the rack and position it above nipple level.

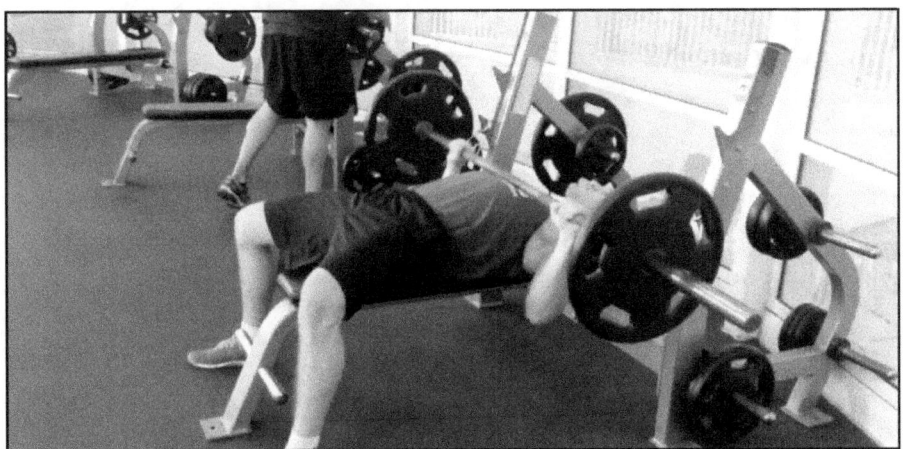

4. Inhale and lower it down until it touches your t-shirt just below your nipples.

5. Exhale and push it back up.

Common Mistakes:

1. Flaring your elbows out to the sides and shrugging your shoulders (touching the bar below your nipples at the bottom will prevent this).

2. Not using a spotter (you don't want to die, have your buddy spot you or man up and ask a stranger at the gym for help).

Alternatives:

1. Dumbbell Chest Press

2. Incline Barbell Chest Press

3. Inclince Dumbbell Chest Press

4. Weighted Push-Ups

5. The Row

Preferred Exercise: Barbell Bent Over Row

Primary Muscles Worked: Back, Biceps, Rear Shoulders

Why:

This is the best back exercise a man can do. It hits virtually every back muscle and will build a thick, manly back. Not to mention, it will crush your biceps as well.

How:

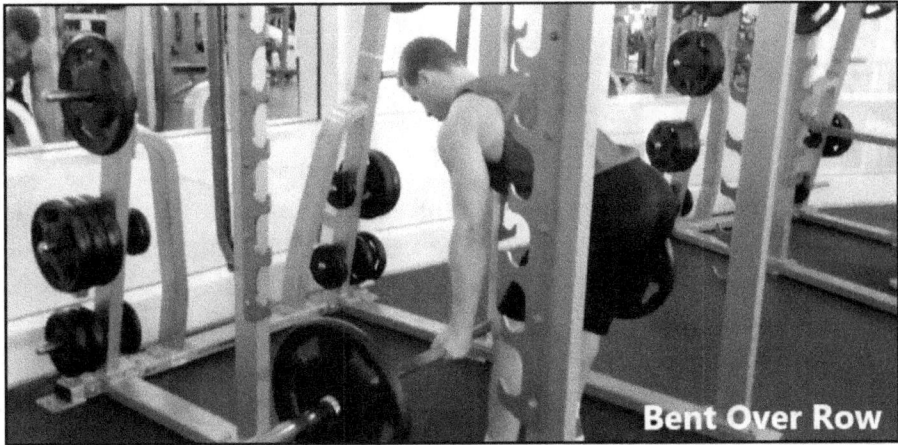

Bent Over Row

1. Grab the barbell with a grip just wider than hip width and lift it from the rack (you can use an over or under hand grip, try both and see what feels more natural).

2. With a slight bend in your knees and keeping your abs tight, lean forward at the hips so that your arms hang straight down and the bar is just below your knees (this is nearly the same position as the bottom of the Romanian Deadlift).

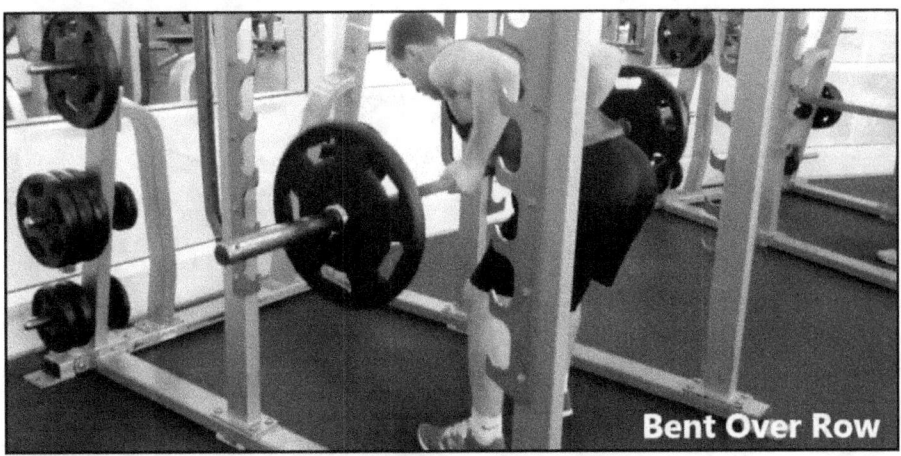

Bent Over Row

3. Exhale and pull the bar up, driving your elbows back and squeezing your shoulder blades together at the top.

31

4. Inhale and lower the bar back down.

Common Mistakes:

1. Standing too upright (make sure you're bent over at the hips at least at a 45 degree angle).

2. Not allowing the bar to travel a full range of motion (your arms should be completely straight at the bottom and your shoulder blades should be completely pinched at the top).

Alternatives:

1. Weighted Pull-Ups

2. Weighted Chin-Ups

3. Seated Cable Row

4. Lat Pulldown

Chapter 7

The Top 6 Accessory Lifts

The five movements I just shared are the foundation for every bodybuilder or strongman's physique and strength. But it doesn't hurt to have a handful of accessory movements to round out the edges.

The following six exercise types will focus on the beach muscles: arms (biceps and triceps), shoulders (side and rear deltoids, the front of the deltoid is already worked extensively by the five big movements), and abdominals.

These muscles are all already worked to some degree by the five big movements, but for optimal development, a little extra work is necessary. The good news is that they're all far easier to execute, so I'll spend less time explaining the form.

1. Triceps

Preferred Exercise: Close Grip Bench Press

Follow the same steps that you would to complete a regular bench press (as described in the previous chapter), only this time grab the bar with a closer grip (just inside of shoulder width apart).

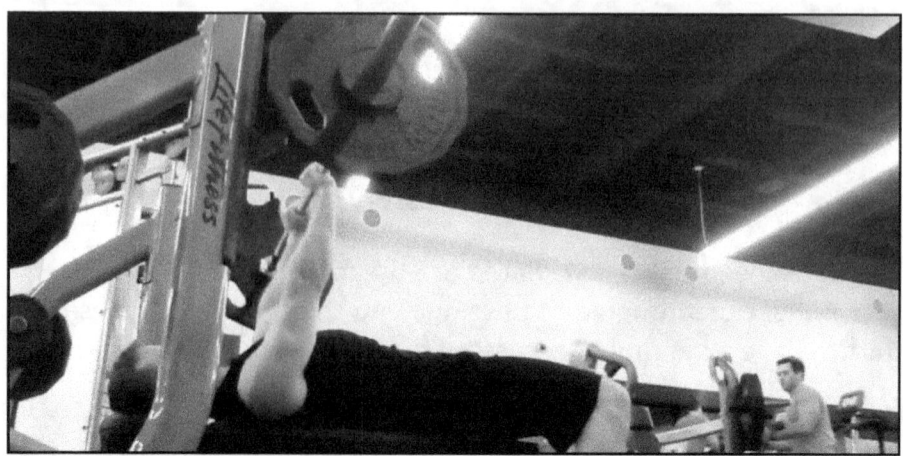

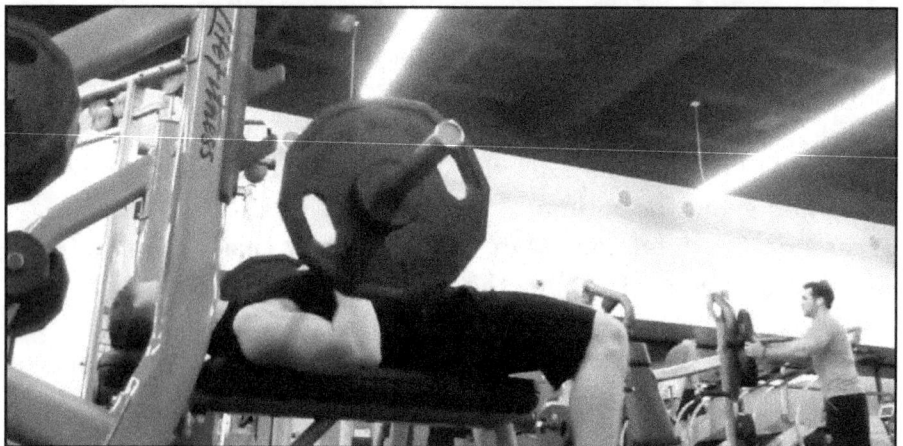

Alternatives:

1. Dumbbell Skull Crushers

2. Barbell Skull Crushers

3. Cable Pulldown

2. Biceps

Preferred Exercise: Barbell Curl

Exhale and curl the barbell up towards your chest, then inhale and drop it back down all the way until your arms are straight. Keep your elbows in place and tight against your ribcage.

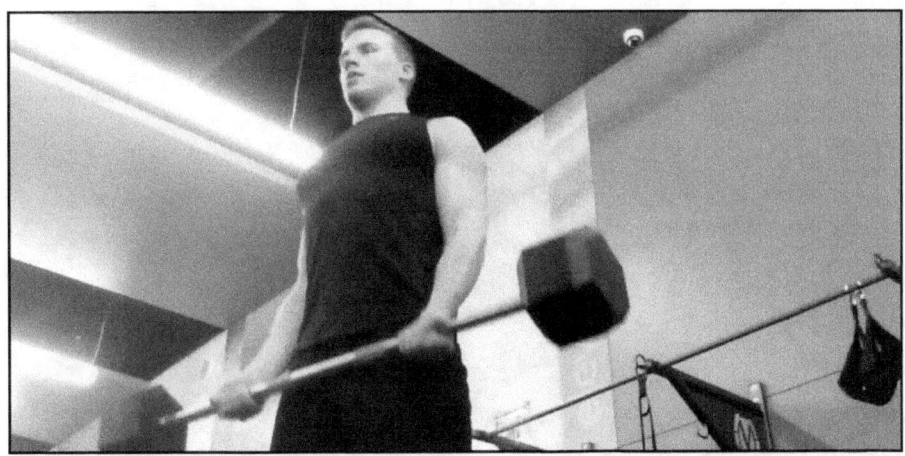

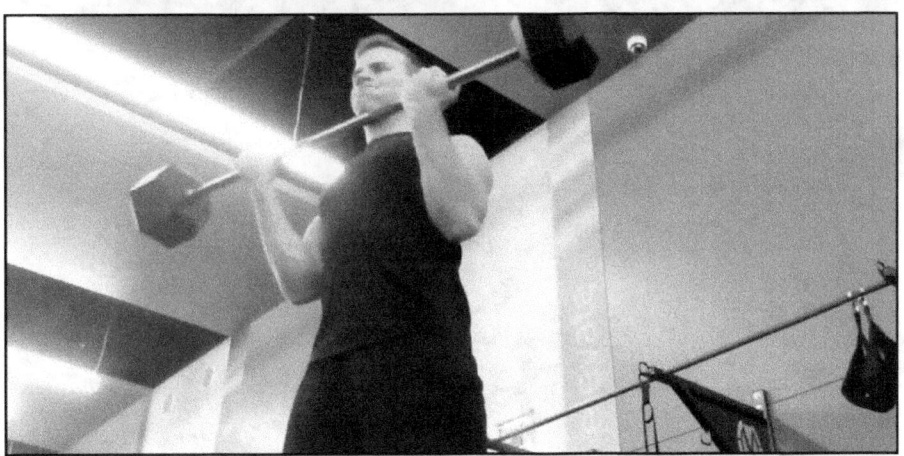

Alternatives:

1. Dumbbell Curl

2. Seated Dumbbell Curl

3. Lateral Deltoid (Side Shoulder)

Preferred Exercise: Lateral Dumbbell Raises

With a slight bend in each arm, exhale and raise your arms up to about shoulder level. Then inhale and drop them back down to your sides.

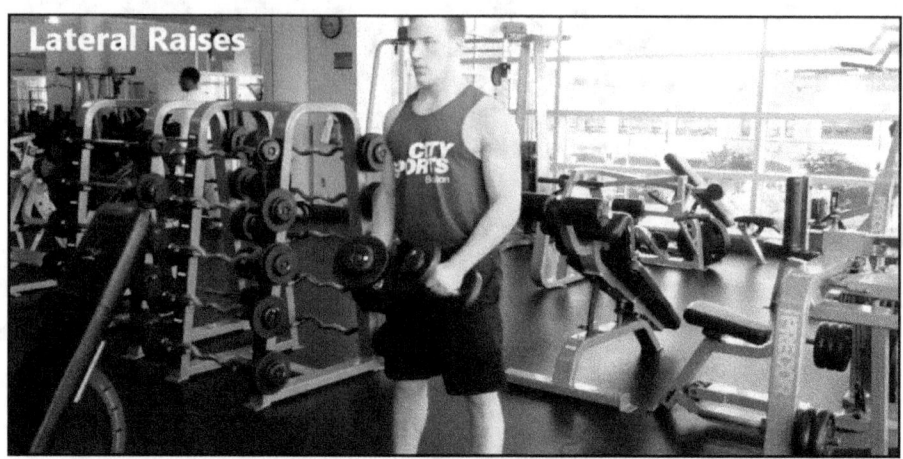

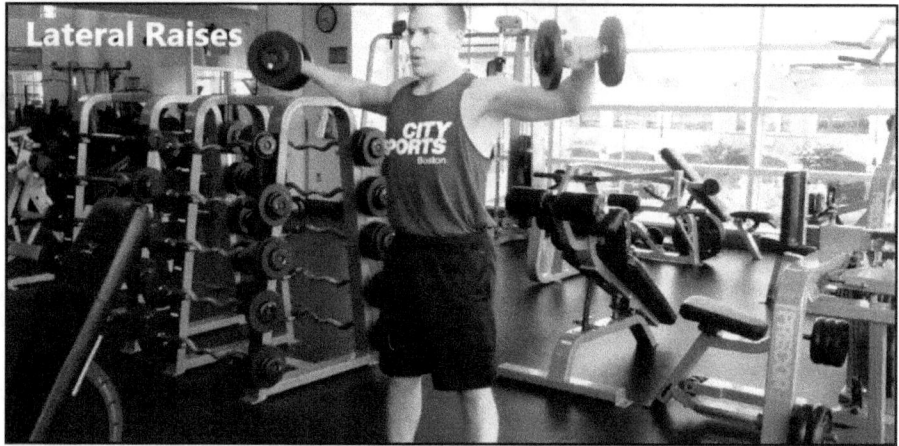

4. Posterior Deltoid (Rear Shoulder)

Preferred Exercise: Lying Rear Dumbbell Raises

Lying face down on an incline bench and holding 2 dumbbells with a slight bend in each arm – exhale and raise your arms up and out to the sides, squeezing your shoulder blades together at the top. Then inhale and return to the starting position.

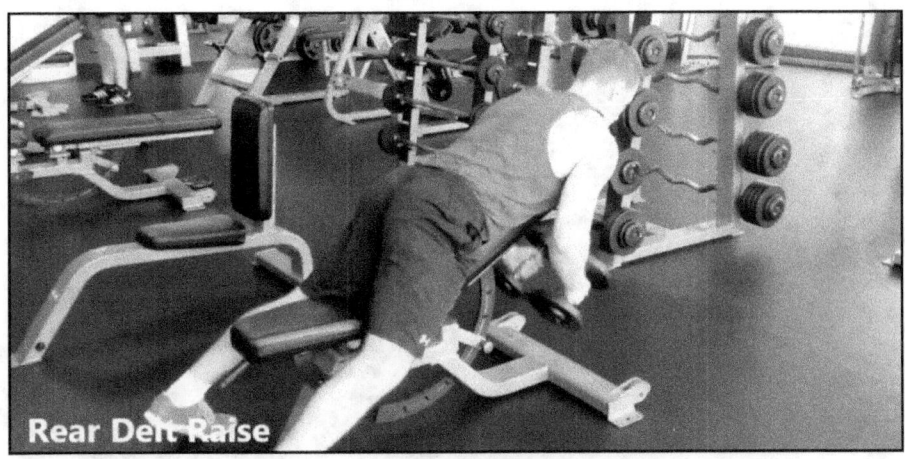

Rear Delt Raise

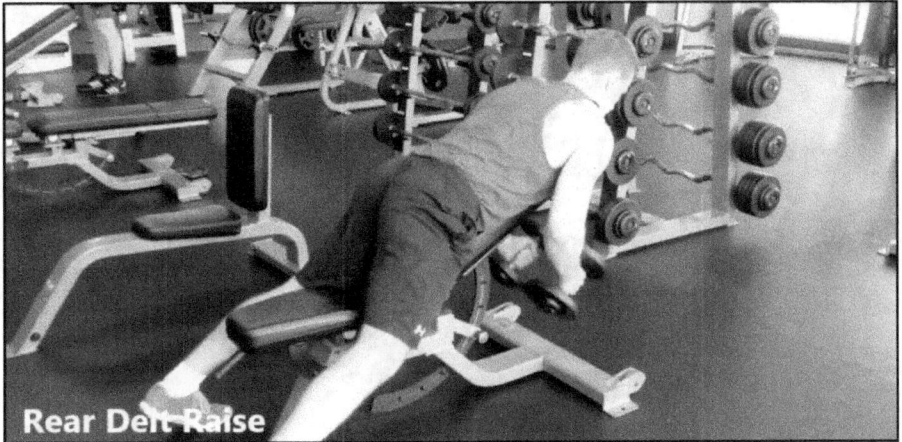

Rear Delt Raise

Alternative:

1. Face Pulls

5. Abdominals

Primary Exercise: Decline Sit-Ups

Seated in a decline sit up bench – inhale and lower your body down until your back barely touches the bench. Then exhale and come back up (the bending should occur at the hips, NOT the middle of the back). Hold a dumbbell in your hands to add difficulty.

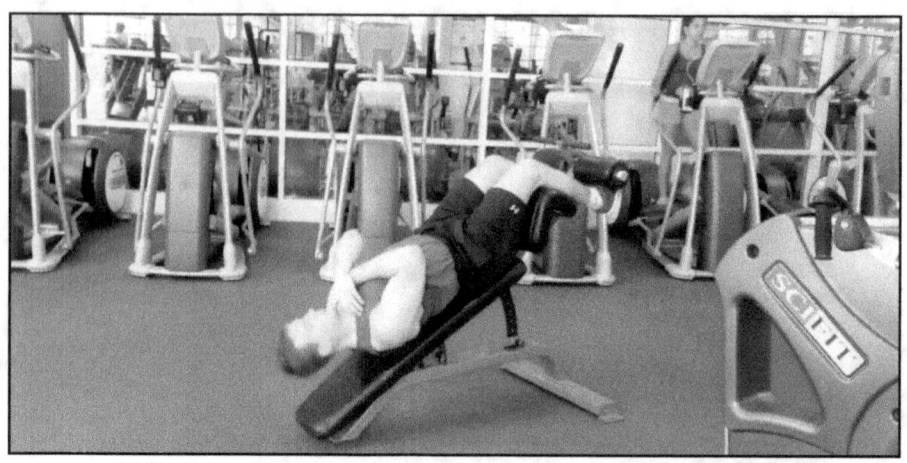

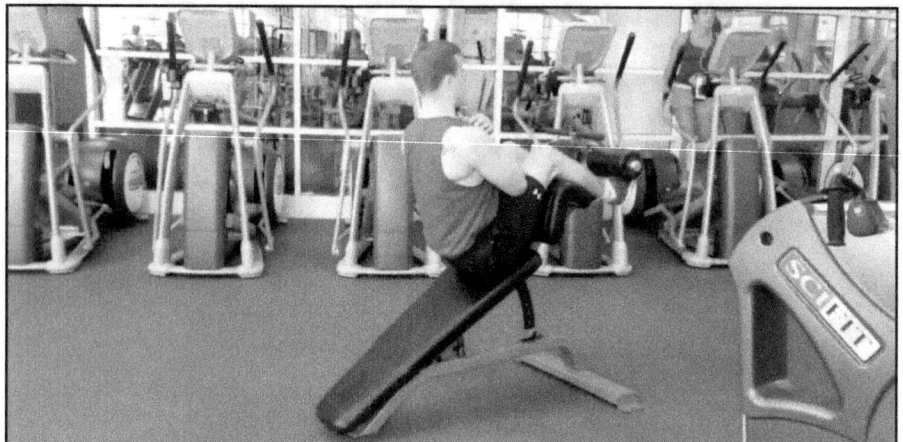

Preferred Exercise 2: Hanging Leg Raises

Hanging from a pull up bar with your legs straight below, exhale and raise your legs up to at least a 90 degree angle. Then inhale and slowly lower them back down.

Note: You can use a leg raises station with a back support if this is too difficult.

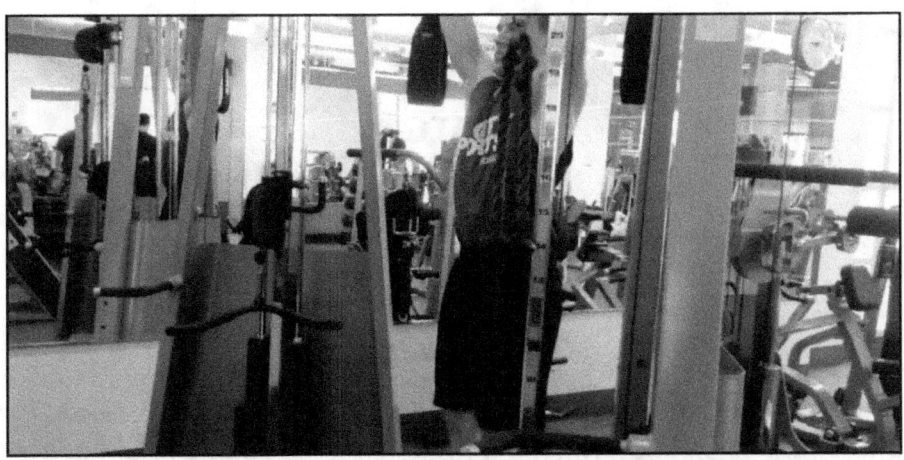

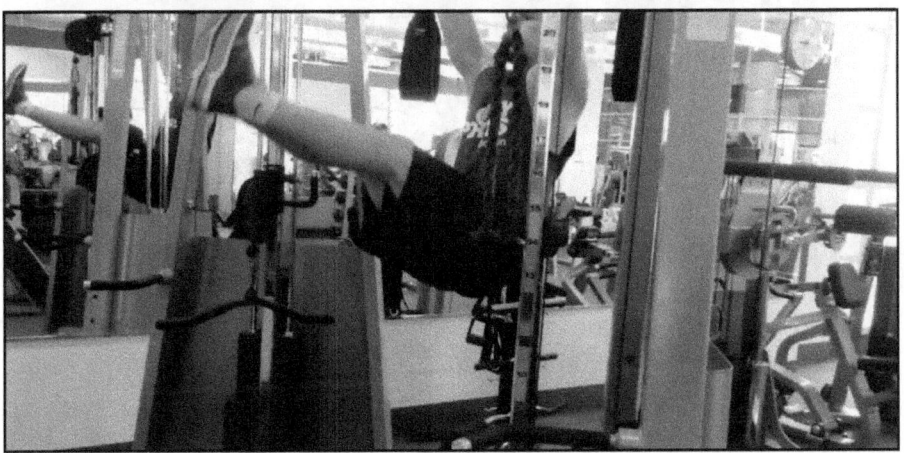

Alternatives:

1. Plank

2. Side Plank

3. Ab Wheel Rollout

4. Cable Reverse Wood-Chop

5. Knee Raises

6. Sit-Ups

Chapter 8

What is the Ideal Male Body?

This is a chapter I decided to include after quite a bit of deliberation.

And I don't mean to force my ideals upon you.

But before we get into the meat of the *Shredded Beast* program, I want to get something out of my system. Something I've undoubtedly hinted at throughout the previous pages of this book. It revolves around the issue of body dysmorphic disorder, or body dysmorphia.

Body dysmorphia is a chronic mental illness where an individual becomes terminally obsessed and unsatisfied with their body. They see imaginary flaws, stare at their bodies in the mirror for unworldly amounts of time, have generally low self-esteem, and commonly suffer from depression as a result.

In the past this has been a problem largely relegated to women, but in recent years, and with the social rise of bodybuilding, it's extended itself to men. There are countless guys out there who start with the best of intentions, to improve their body, but then end up ruining themselves instead.

It most commonly happens with guys who want to get *ripped* or *shredded*. They go through a period of fat loss, look great, and then instead of stopping and being happy or switching their focus to building muscle, they strive for lower and lower body fat percentages.

They get so caught up in their own little world that they completely lose touch with reality.

1. Being anywhere below 8% body fat is unhealthy. And the caloric deficit needed to get there takes a large toll on your body.

2. To get to that level of leanness, you can eat barely any food. Food will cease to be a source of pleasure.

3. It doesn't look good. Being insanely lean looks girly — women don't find it attractive and men don't respect it.

Get to the point, already.

I bring up this issue because Phase 1 of the *Shredded Beast* program is a period of fat loss.

It's meant to get you down to an acceptable level of body fat, from which you can enjoy food and focus on getting stronger, without worrying about getting fat.

The thing is an acceptable level of body fat means something completely different to all of us. I just want to make sure that no one goes overboard and gets obsessed with fat loss, because of the dangers I mentioned above.

I find that the best level of body fat to maintain year-round is when your abs are visible, but only when flexed. You look great naked, but can still enjoy food and not constantly worry about "losing your six pack." This is the level I encourage you to aim for during Phase 1 of the *Shredded Beast* program. It will put you in a great place to focus on building muscle, getting stronger, and being a man.

The only reason to get shredded beyond this point is if you're a bodybuilder about to hop on stage or a model getting ready for a photo-shoot.

Chapter 9

How to Build and Customize Your Personal *Shredded Beast* Training Plan

I've already shared which exercises I believe are best, but I won't dictate exactly what you should do.

Everyone is different. We all operate under different circumstances. Maybe you don't have access to a full gym with a squat rack. Maybe an injury you've suffered prevents you from doing specific exercises. In this chapter we'll construct a program that's custom-tailored to suit your unique needs and preferences.

The *Shredded Beast* program relies on alternating between two weight lifting routines. Both of these routines will hit your whole body, albeit with slightly different focuses. Your job is to choose exercises from chapters 6 and 7 to pair with each movement type I've listed below. I've included example choices in parenthesis. These are the preferred exercises (when in doubt – use them).

Day One Routine

1. **Squat** (e.g. barbell box squat)

2. **Overhead Press** (e.g. barbell standing shoulder press)

3. **Pull** (e.g. barbell bent-over rows)

4. **Triceps** (e.g. close grip bench press)

5. **Rear Deltoid** (e.g. lying rear shoulder raises)

6. **Abs** (e.g. decline sit-ups)

Day Two Routine

1. **Squat** (e.g. barbell box squat)

2. **Deadlift** (e.g. Romanian deadlift)

3. **Chest Press** (e.g. barbell bench press)

4. **Pull** (e.g. weighted pull ups)

5. **Biceps** (e.g. barbell curls)

6. **Lateral Deltoid** (e.g. dumbbell lateral raises)

7. **Abs** (e.g. hanging leg raises)

Note: For my example I chose to use the same squat exercise (box squats) for both days. You can do this or select different ones for each day. The same goes for the pull exercises.

Once you've written down your selections, keep reading to see how you'll put this plan into action.

Chapter 10

Shredded Beast Phase 1: The Shred

Gentlemen, welcome to the *Shredded Beast* training program. We'll begin with Phase 1.

The Objective

The objective of this phase is to *cut fat until you reach a level of leanness acceptable to you*.

Keep in mind: this should not be the body fat levels of a fitness model or competitive bodybuilder, because the effort and dietary restriction is takes to get to there is unhealthy and the end result isn't manly.

This phase is meant to create your base physique, from which you'll add strength and muscle indefinitely, while remaining lean and athletic.

If you're already at a body fat level that's acceptable to you, and you want to focus on building muscle and getting stronger, then skip ahead to Phase 2 (chapter 11).

The Diet

Your dietary goal is to lose one pound per week. If you follow the steps below in addition to the training protocol laid out on the coming pages, this weight loss will be all, or nearly all, fat loss (as opposed to muscle loss).

1. Calculate your estimated caloric intake needed to lose fat using the steps provided in Chapter 4.

2. Calculate your protein needs (.75 grams per pound of body

weight).

3. Keep a rough estimate of your daily caloric intake using an app like *Calorie Counter* by *FatSecret*. Aim for the number you calculated in step 1.

4. Weigh yourself every two weeks (in the morning, after using the bathroom, but before eating). If you're losing around one pound per week, keep it up. If you're not losing weight, subtract 200 calories from your target daily caloric intake.

...or skip these steps and follow *The Lazy Man's Approach to Losing Weight* from chapter 4.

In chapters 19 and 20 I'll share a list of foods and meals I recommend to help you achieve this goal.

The Training

Your training goal is to gain or maintain strength. This will guarantee that your weight loss is primarily fat, and that you maintain your muscle mass (and possibly even gain some muscle).

You'll alternate between the two routines you created in chapter 9, performing them on three non-consecutive weekdays.

Example: Day 1 on Monday, Day 2 on Wednesday, Day 1 on Friday, Day 2 on Monday, etc.

Yes, you're only lifting three days per week — this is because you're working out your entire body each time you go. For a full explanation of why this is preferable to working out five or six days per week and doing different muscles each time, see chapter 16.

You're also not doing an awful lot of volume (the total number of sets and reps — you won't be in the gym that long over the course of the week). This is because when you're losing weight you don't have the energy to be in the gym for an hour every day of the week (literally — you're in a caloric deficit). It will only lead to burn-out and an overstressed nervous system.

Day One Routine

1. Squat: 3x5

2. Overhead Press: 3x5

3. Pull: 3x5

4. Triceps: 2x8

5. Rear Deltoid: 2x8

6. Abs: 2x8

Day Two Routine

1. Squat: 2x5

2. Deadlift: 1x5

3. Chest Press: 3x5

4. Pull: 3x5

5. Biceps: 2x8

6. Lateral Deltoid: 2x8

7. Abs: 2x8

Starting Weights

Choose starting weights that you know you can execute the prescribed number of sets and reps with. If you're unsure, or the exercises are brand new to you, then choose light weights. Don't worry — you'll quickly increase the weights as you go.

Warm Up

To warm up perform the flexibility routine included in chapter 13. Also do one warm up set for the first three exercises each day with 50% of the weight you'll be using.

Rest Periods

Rest 2-3 minutes in between sets of the 5 rep exercises (the first three you perform each day) and 60-90 seconds in between sets of the 8 rep variety (the last three you perform each day).

Repetition Tempo

For every exercise: lower the weight slowly and under control (1-2 seconds) and lift it quickly (0-1 seconds). This ensures you're using a manageable weight with good form, and also builds explosive power.

The Progression

Getting stronger is far more difficult when you're losing weight, because your body is in a caloric deficit – it has less energy than it needs to maintain.

However, with a good deal of focus and effort, I believe you can and will get stronger. Follow this progression to do so efficiently:

1. If you complete the prescribed number of sets and repetitions for a given exercise, add 5 pounds the next time you do that exercise.

Example: Box Squats, 185 pounds, 3x5 →next time you will use 190 pounds

2. If you fail to complete all of the prescribed number of sets and repetitions for a given exercise, subtract 10% of the weight the next time you do that exercise.

Example: Box Squats, 185 pounds, 2x5, 1x3 (failed on the last set) →

next time you will use 165 pounds

By following this progression you'll add strength at a consistent rate. The 10% drops in weight will happen often, and this is intentional. By always dropping the weight when you fail, you'll be able to build back up and push through plateaus.

Most guys keep pounding away when they hit a strength wall. This leads to burn-out. By taking a step back, your body can recover so that when you work your way back up to where you failed before, it's ready to crush it and get stronger.

For Exercises That Don't Use Weights

You might have included an exercise that doesn't use weights as part of your routine (e.g. push-ups, pull-ups, sit-ups, leg raises, etc.). If you cannot perform the prescribed amount of reps with one of these, then do as many as possible.

If you can do more than the prescribed number of reps, then add weight (by using a weighted vest, backpack, or holding a dumbbell in between your legs). If you can't figure out a way to add weight, then do as many reps as you can.

The Cardio

Perform 2 days of cardio per week during Phase 1 to assist in your fat loss efforts. See chapter 15 for my opinion on what type of cardio is best.

Chapter 11

Shredded Beast Phase 2: The Beast

Most of your time (over the course of your fitness career) should be aimed at getting stronger and building muscle.

Getting and staying reasonably lean is important, yes, but pushing to make improvements in the gym is the basis of any sustainable program that will lead to not only the strongest, but also the best looking body in the long run.

This is the guiding principle of Phase 2, where you'll be performing the bulk of your work. Begin Phase 2 once you're at an acceptable level of body fat and you're ready to focus on building muscle and getting stronger.

The Objective

The objective is to build muscle and get stronger. You'll aim to surpass your previous best every time you're in the gym.

The Diet

Your dietary goal is to maintain or slightly increase your weight as you go.

You don't want to put on more than half a pound per week, because the body isn't capable of synthesizing more muscle tissue naturally (if you're on steroids, then you bought the wrong book).

You'll be doing a higher volume of training, so it's important that you eat enough to at least maintain your weight as you go. Your body needs the fuel.

1. Calculate your estimated caloric intake needed to gain muscle

using the steps provided in Chapter 4.

2. Calculate your protein needs (.75 grams per pound of body weight).

3. Keep a rough estimate of your daily caloric intake using an app like *Calorie Counter* by *FatSecret*. Aim for the number you calculated in step 1.

4. Weigh yourself every two weeks (in the morning, after using the bathroom, but before eating). If you're maintaining or losing weight, add 200 calories per day to achieve a slight caloric surplus.

...or skip these steps and follow *The Lazy Man's Approach to Gaining Weight* from chapter 4.

In chapters 19 and 20 I'll share a list of foods and meals I recommend to help you achieve this goal.

The Training

Your training goal is simple: get stronger.

Achieving this goal will guarantee that most, if not all of the weight you gain will be in the form of muscle mass (as opposed to fat).

Similarly to Phase 1, you'll alternate between the two routines you created in chapter 9, performing them on three non-consecutive weekdays.

Example: Day 1 on Monday, Day 2 on Wednesday, Day 1 on Friday, Day 2 on Monday, etc.

Yes, you're only lifting three days per week – this is because you're working out your entire body each time you go. For a full explanation of why this is preferable to working out five or six days per week and doing different muscles each time, see chapter 16.

You'll notice you're doing the same workouts as in Phase 1, except with a lot more volume (sets and reps). This is on purpose. The added volume will take advantage of the extra calories you're consuming. If you want further variety in exercise selection, hold off for now – I'll cover this topic in the next chapter.

Day One Routine

1. Squat: 5x5

2. Overhead Press: 5x5

3. Pull: 5x5

4. Triceps: 3x8

5. Rear Deltoid: 3x8

6. Abs: 3x8

Day Two Routine

1. Squat: 3x5

2. Deadlift: 2x5

3. Chest Press: 5x5

4. Pull: 5x5

5. Biceps: 3x8

6. Lateral Deltoid: 3x8

7. Abs: 3x8

Starting Weights

Choose starting weights that you know you can execute the

prescribed number of sets and reps with. If you're unsure, or the exercises are brand new to you, then choose light weights. Don't worry – you'll quickly increase the weights as you go.

Warm Up

To warm up perform the flexibility routine included in chapter 13. Also do one warm up set for the first three exercises each day with 50% of the weight you'll be using.

Rest Periods

Rest 2-3 minutes in between sets of the 5 rep exercises (the first three you perform each day) and 60-90 seconds in between sets of the 8 rep variety (the last three you perform each day).

Repetition Tempo

For every exercise: lower the weight slowly and under control (1-2 seconds) and lift it quickly (0-1 seconds). This ensures you're using a manageable weight with good form, and also builds explosive power.

The Progression

Remember, lifting more and more weight is the goal of Phase 2.

We'll be using the same progression from Phase 1 to accomplish this, but you should be able to make more progress without having to reset, because of your increased caloric intake.

1. If you complete the prescribed number of sets and repetitions for a given exercise, add 5 pounds the next time you do that exercise.

Example: Box Squats, 185 pounds, 5x5 →next time you will use 190 pounds

2. If you fail to complete all of the prescribed number of sets and repetitions for a given exercise, subtract 10% of the weight the next

time you do that exercise.

Example: Box Squats, 185 pounds, 4x5, 1x3 (failed on the last set) → *next time you will use 165 pounds*

By following this progression you'll add strength at a consistent rate. The 10% drops in weight will happen often, and this is intentional. By always dropping the weight when you fail, you'll be able to build back up and push through plateaus.

Most guys keep pounding away when they hit a strength wall. This leads to burn-out. By taking a step back, your body can recover so that when you work your way back up to where you failed before, it's ready to crush it and get stronger.

For Exercises That Don't Use Weights

You might have included an exercise that doesn't use weights as part of your routine (e.g. push-ups, pull-ups, sit-ups, leg raises, etc.). If you cannot perform the prescribed amount of reps with one of these, then do as many as possible.

If you can do more than the prescribed number of reps, then add weight (by using a weighted vest, backpack, or holding a dumbbell in between your feet). If you can't figure out a way to add weight, then do as many reps as you can.

The Cardio

Perform 1 day of cardio per week during Phase 2 to maintain the benefits it offers while keeping your focus on the weights. See chapter 15 for my opinion on what type of cardio is best.

You're free to do more if you want, but realize that you may have to eat more to make up for the additional energy you expend during bouts of cardio to ensure proper recovery.

Chapter 12

How to Maintain the Body of a *Shredded Beast*

Now that you've seen both parts of the *Shredded Beast* program, it's time to look at how to apply them over the long haul.

For the most part, follow this simple rule: use Phase 1 any time that you feel uncomfortably fat, and use Phase 2 the rest of the time.

This will result in the best possible physique. You'll be adding muscle (Phase 2) the vast majority of the time. Then, at any point that you feel you've put on a bit too much belly fat along with the muscle, you'll switch over to cutting fat (Phase 1) and reveal your newly added muscle in the process.

But don't switch back and forth too frequently

It takes time to remove a significant portion of excess fat, and even more time to build a measurable amount of muscle. For this reason I advise the following minimums:

1. Dedicate at least 1 continuous month at a time to successfully complete a Phase 1.

2. Dedicate at least 3 continuous months at a time to successfully complete a Phase 2.

If you want to go longer than those timeframes, that's fine. You just want to avoid the trap of switching back and forth every few weeks. This will drive you mentally crazy and be terribly inefficient as well.

If you get bored of some of the exercises

Feel free to swap out any of the accessory movements (exercises 4-6 of each day) for alternatives you like that, and also hit the same muscles. However, don't do this too frequently. Stick with accessory movements for at least one month at a time.

In regards to the core lifts (exercises 1-3 of each day), stick with them for at least three months at a time. These are the bread and butter of any good athlete, bodybuilder, or powerlifter's training program. Getting stronger in these lifts is what will get you results, so get used to doing them for longer periods of time.

Follow the guidelines I set forth here and you'll see drastic improvements in your physique over the next few months and years. That's a promise.

Chapter 13

A Simple Yet Effective Stretching Routine

Stretching is the bane of every man's existence. Well, that and filing taxes. It just seems to useless and boring. But it's not. Not useless, that is. It's still pretty boring.

The top three reasons you should stretch are:

1. Increased flexibility and joint range of motion

2. Improved posture

3. Reduced risk of injury

Luckily I have a nifty little routine that will make it quick and painless, and also double as a good warm up. This is crucial because it forces you to stretch bit each time you work out – no more forgetting.

Perform the following eight moves every time before you work out. They focus on lower body and hip mobility, because that's where most guys struggle. All you need is a foam roller and about five minutes.

Note: Full credit for the following routine goes to Joe DeFranco of **www.defrancostraining.com**.

1. Foam Roll IT Band (30 seconds per side)

Position yourself on your side with the foam roller beneath your lower leg. Roll down to the knee and up to the hip. Go slowly and rest on any trigger points (tender spots) for 10 seconds.

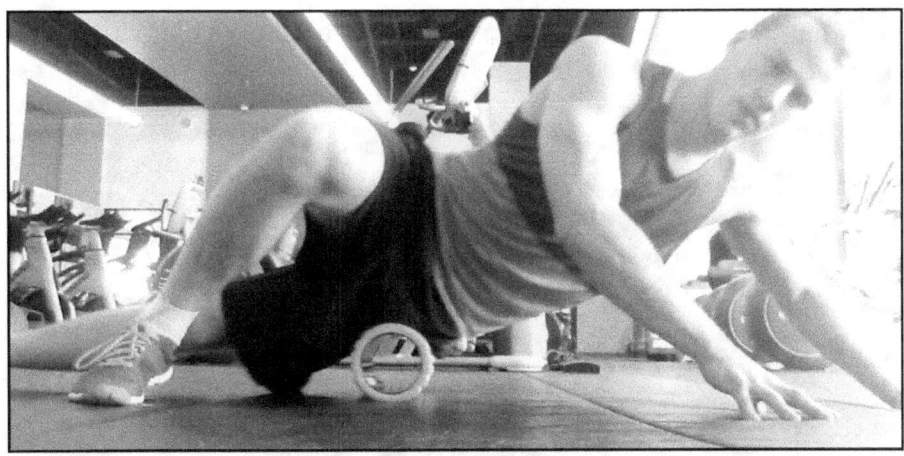

2. Foam Roll Piriformis/Glutes (30 seconds per side)

Position yourself seated on the foam roller and cross one leg over the opposite knee. Roll the upper butt/lower back area of the side whose leg is crossed over. Go slowly and rest on any trigger points (tender spots) for 10 seconds.

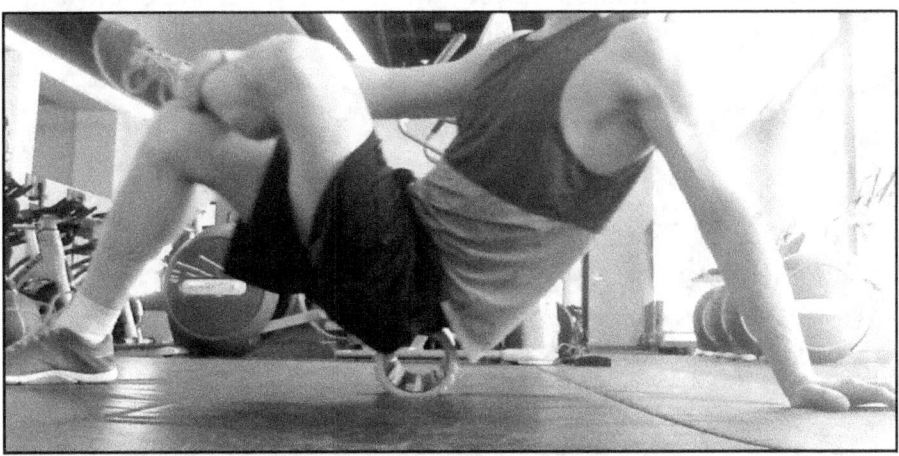

3. Foam Roll Adductors (30 seconds per side)

Position yourself prone on top of the foam roller with one leg straight behind you and the other bent at a 90 degree angle and on top of the foam roller. Using your elbows, roll back and forth between the knee and the groin. Go slowly and rest on any trigger points (tender spots) for 10 seconds.

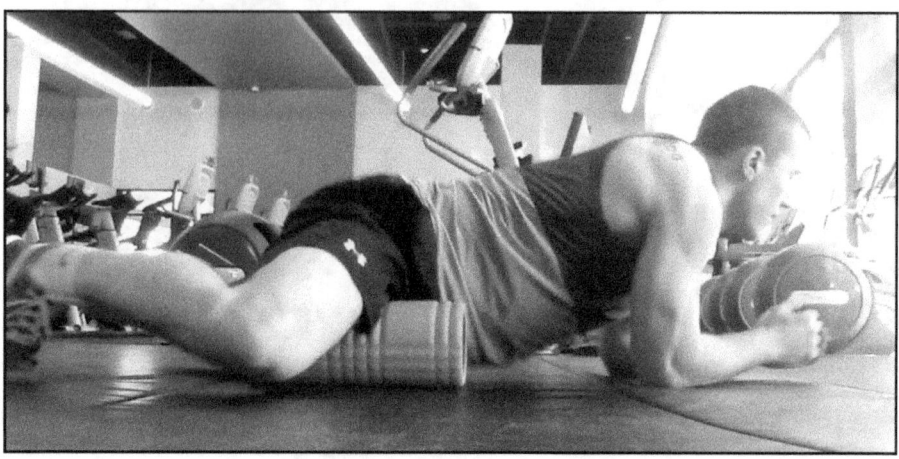

4. Rollovers into V-Sits (10 reps)

Sit down and then fall back, allowing your feet to come overhead and touch the ground behind you, then roll forward and end with your legs spread apart and your hands touching your toes.

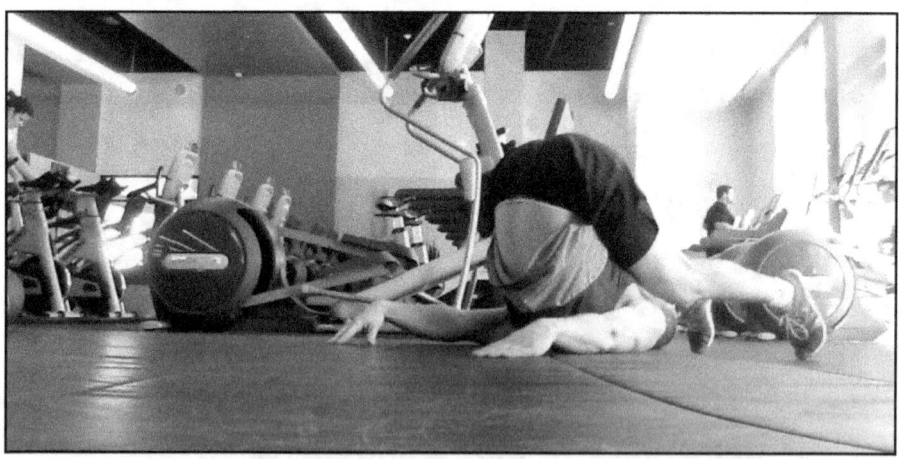

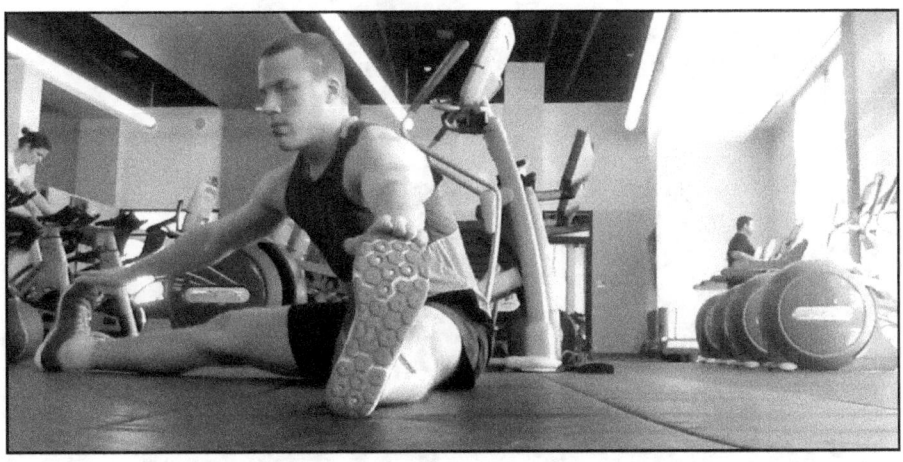

5. Fire Hydrants (10 forward circles/10 backward circles per side)

Position yourself facing down on your hands and knees. Then lift one knee from the floor and make ten big circles, bringing your knee all the way up to your chest, out to the side, and then back behind you. Then switch directions and make ten big circles going the opposite direction.

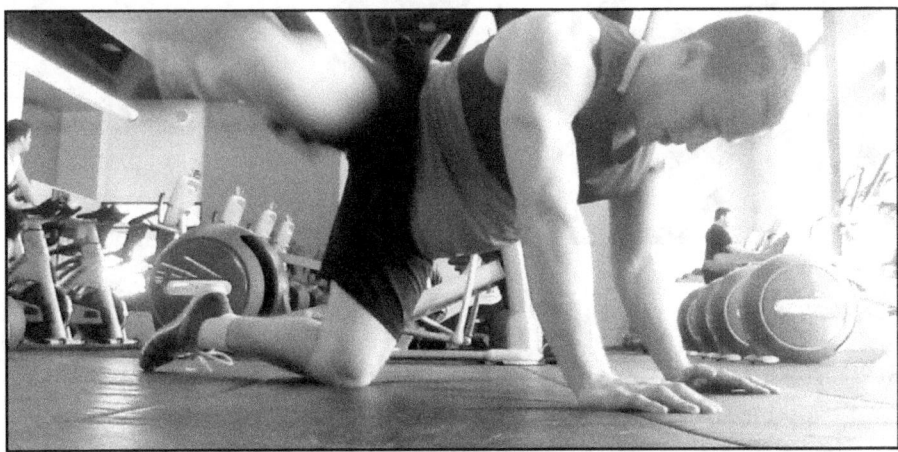

6. Mountains Climbers (20 reps)

Start in a push up position with one foot outside of and next to the hand on the same side of your body. Then jump and switch, bringing that foot back and the other foot forward to the other hand.

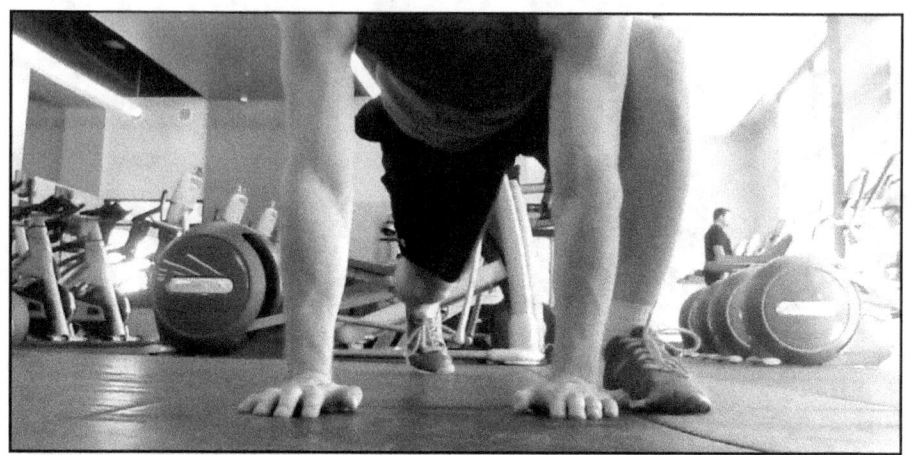

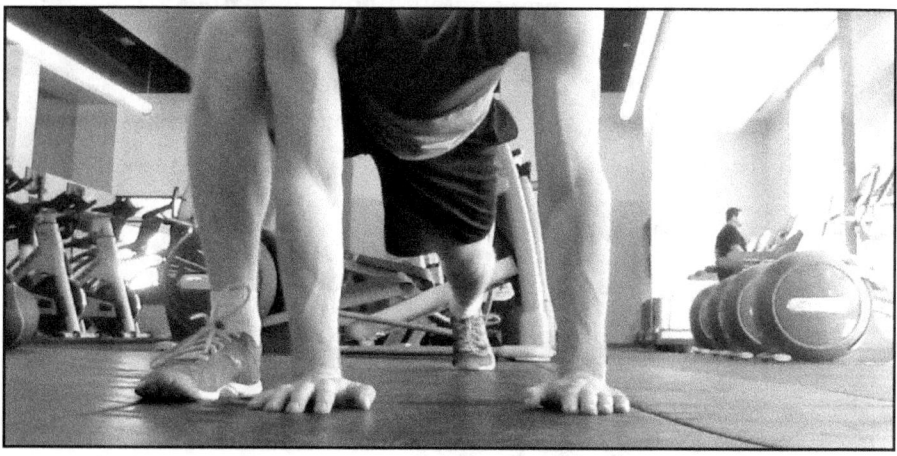

7. Groiners (10 reps)

Start in a push up position and then jump both hands forward so that they land outside of your hands. Then jump back to the push up position.

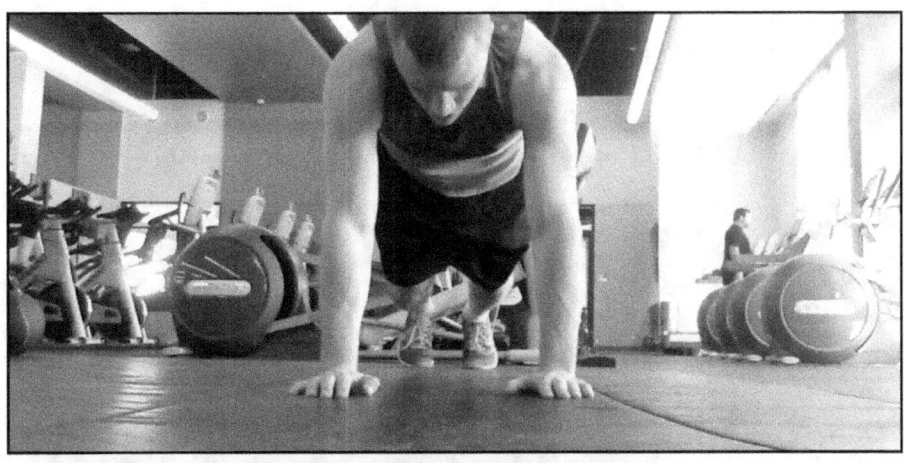

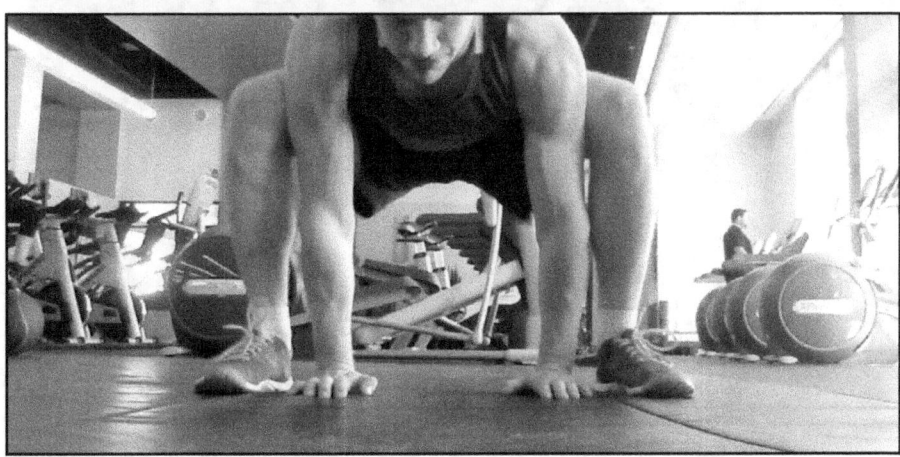

8. Hip Flexor Stretch (3 sets of 10 seconds per leg)

Kneeling with your torso upright, lean forward so that you feel a stretch next to the groin, where your leg meets your hip.

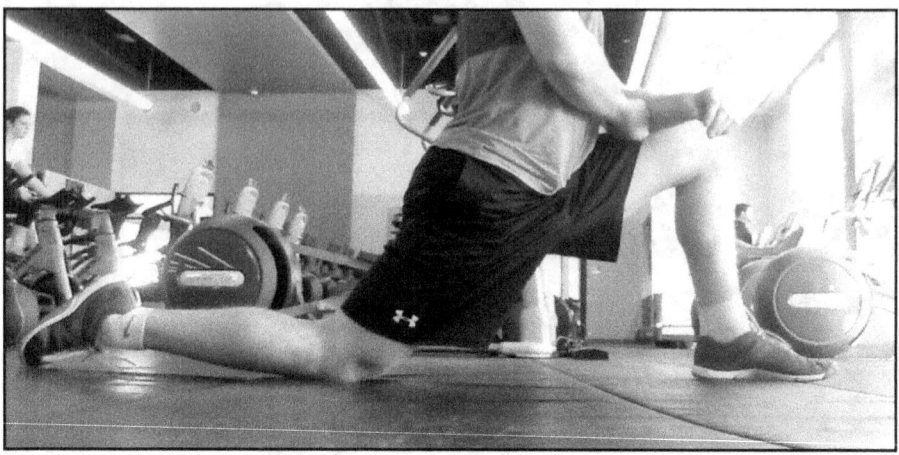

Chapter 14

Why Supplements are a Waste of Money

That's right. I don't use them.

It's not long ago that I did. But over the last year I've taken the red pill and seen the truth:

Supplements don't do shit for you.

I'm going to break the most popular supplements down one by one, and tell you why you don't need them.

1. Multivitamins

Long hailed as a cornerstone of the American diet, these pills' actual effectiveness has been called into question recently.

In late 2013, a trio of studies conducted by researchers at Johns Hopkins, the University of Warwick, and the American College of Physicians were released in the *Annals of Internal Medicine*.

What did they find?

In conclusion, β-carotene, vitamin E, and possibly high doses of vitamin A supplements are harmful. Other antioxidants, folic acid and B vitamins, and multivitamin and mineral supplements are ineffective for preventing mortality or morbidity due to major chronic diseases. Although available evidence does not rule out small benefits or harms or large benefits or harms in a small subgroup of the population, we believe that the case is closed— **supplementing the diet of well-nourished adults with (most) mineral or vitamin supplements has no clear benefit and might even be harmful**. *These vitamins should not be used for chronic* *disease prevention. Enough is enough.* (20)

No cloudy words or unclear results are found here. The authors of these studies firmly believe that multivitamins have been proven ineffective, and even potentially harmful to your health.

The release of these studies led to an inevitable backlash from the supplement industry and other doctors, all in support of multivitamins. And quite honestly – I'm not sure who to believe. There's conflicting evidence out there.

The one thing I *am* sure of is that the best route we can all take is to eat a varied diet that includes fruits and vegetables. Yes, I sound like your grandmother, but it's true. It's the only way to guarantee that you'll properly ingest all of the nutrients your body needs to thrive.

2. Pre-workout Powder

This shit has been flying off the shelves of your local GNC for the past few years. At least 90% of guys ages 18-30 I know who lift weights take this stuff.

Hell, even I do from time to time.

Why? Because it makes you feel like an absolute monster. Seriously, it makes you believe that you could put the whole world on your shoulders – and then squat it four or five times. But guess what. It doesn't do shit. I can lift just as much weight as I can with a pre-workout drink, without one. All it does it make you *feel* like a boss.

Read their marketing campaigns and product labels. They promote increased energy and focus, not added muscle or reduced fat. Not even more strength. And this truth boils down to one very basic fact: the active ingredient in the vast majority of pre-workout supplements is caffeine. That's right, the same thing that you get in a standard cup of morning joe.

From time to time you'll see one get banned. And it's always because it had something stronger inside: a more intense stimulant.

So next time you need that pre-workout push, go for some coffee instead. It's cheaper, more natural, and doesn't contain one hundred extra ingredients you've never heard of (and can't even pronounce).

Better yet, just push through your fatigue and be a man. One good set of heavy squats or rows will have you buzzing like a bee.

3. Creatine

Creatine is an organic acid, naturally synthesized by our bodies from several amino acids, that helps to supply energy to the cells of the body, especially in skeletal muscle.

It has the ability to rapidly regenerate ATP (adenosine triphosphate). This assists in sustaining high intensity muscular efforts for up to 10 seconds.

Supplementing creatine while lifting weights ensures high levels of the acid in the body, and has been shown to increase muscle mass and improve strength. It's normal to gain 4 to 5 pounds when beginning supplementation, as creatine causes as osmotic effect that draws more water into the muscles (27).

But I still don't recommend taking it. The observed strength increase is minimal, a percentage of the population has been shown to be non-responders (i.e. it doesn't even work for everyone), and it's just one more thing to make sure you take every day.

But it's cheap, so go for it if you really want to.

4. Protein Powder

I'm going to make this very clear: protein powder is a food, not a supplement.

It's just a processed form of protein.

And I'm actually *not* going to tell you not to buy it.

If you have trouble achieving your protein intake goal of 0.75 grams per pound of bodyweight per day, then protein powder is an easy and relatively cheap way to get you there. But it's not required. And hitting that mark is really not difficult with normal food.

So don't be tricked into thinking that downing a couple scoops of protein powder after a workout is going to do something magical.

I can feel my muscle growing already!

No, you can't. I'll explain why in the meal timing chapter.

The 2 Exceptions: Fish Oil and Vitamin D

There are two supplements that I *do* take. I know I'm contradicting myself, but I don't care.

If you don't regularly eat fatty fish (like salmon) then supplementing a few grams of fish oil every day is a good call.

Various studies have shown numerous general health benefits from supplementing fish oil (namely decreased risk of cardiovascular disease). It also has a positive effect on insulin sensitivity, making it potentially helpful for your muscle building goals (21).

The other pill that I pop is vitamin D3. Vitamin D3 is only synthesized by our bodies when we have a solid amount of exposure to the sun. So if you live somewhere where you're not getting exposed to sunlight regularly, then it's a good idea to buy and take a vitamin D3 supplement.

The dangers of incurring a vitamin D3 deficiency are numerous. It's been shown to compromise the immune system and even lead to softening of the bones (22).

Chapter 15

What is the Best Type of Cardio for a Man?

Give me a couple hundred pounds of iron and I'll have a field day. I'll squat it, push it, pull it, pick it up, and then put it back down.

Give me a treadmill or an elliptical and I'll take a nap on it or try to lift it before using it as intended. I said it once and I'll say it again: cardio sucks. But it does have its place.

1. Cardio is good for your health. It strengthens your heart and decreases blood pressure (25).

2. It's also a useful dietary tool when losing weight – you expend more calories when you cycle, swim, or run than when you're resting. This allows you to eat slightly more while still maintaining a caloric deficit. Just realize you're losing weight because of your diet, NOT the cardio.

But even that knowledge isn't enough to get me on a treadmill or elliptical. Now if someone held a family member of mine hostage and would only release them if I did 30 minutes on the stationary bike, then I can see the justification for a little cardio.

Anything short of that and I'm out. There are some types of cardio I can get behind, however.

1. Sports

Men are competitive creatures. We thrive in competitive environments.

Just because you graduated high school doesn't mean you should give up sports. If you can find a good men's basketball or soccer league and you enjoy playing, then you should sign up.

You'll compete, make new man friends, and get a bit of cardio in as an added benefit.

2. Martial Arts

This has been my personal favorite form of cardio over the past few years, and not because I get a cardio workout while training.

I love it because there's nothing more badass or manly than knowing how to fight and defend yourself.

First I took Krav Maga, which is a brutal self-defense system. You don't get to compete fully because elbows to the face and knees to the groin are encouraged. But I now know how to disarm someone with a pistol or a knife and then beat their face in.

Now I'm taking Muay Thai, which *is* a competitive martial art. Again, I do it for the skills I'm learning and the enjoyment it brings me – the cardio is just an added benefit.

3. Hiking/Cycling

The last form of cardio I enjoy is hiking or cycling though nature.

It's definitely a great form of stress relief, and in today's world we simply don't get outside enough. Be a man, explore the wild, and get in a little cardio while you're at it.

Chapter 16

Why Full Body Routines are Superior to Split Routines

The *Shredded Beast* training program is a full body routine. You work every muscle group each time you hit the gym.

The common alternative to this is called a split. An example of a split is chest on Monday, back on Tuesday, legs on Wednesday, shoulders on Thursday, and arms on Friday.

The full body routine is superior to the split. Every man should be doing full body. Here's why.

1. More Frequent Spikes in Muscle Protein Synthesis

As we covered earlier, when you lift weights your rates of muscle protein synthesis are raised for about 36 hours. This is what leads to muscular development and increased strength.

When you do a full body routine you're raising these rates of muscle protein synthesis for your entire body three times per week. When you do a split routine, you're only hitting each body part, and therefore only raising the rates of muscle protein synthesis for those muscles, once or twice a week.

Simple math tells us that three is greater than one (or two). More frequent spikes in muscle protein synthesis will lead to quicker growth and development.

2. More Quality Reps over the Course of the Week

There's one major point of contention every proponent of a split routine will make in response to my above argument. This is that with a split routine, even though you only hit the chest once per week, when you hit it, you hit it hard. Unfortunately, this doesn't lead to equal spikes in muscle protein synthesis over the course of a week.

For example, you might only be targeting your chest with five sets of bench press in a full body workout. On a chest day in a split you would do those five sets of bench press and then follow it up with multiple sets of incline bench press, chest flies, and push-ups – a lot more volume than the five sets of bench press you would've done using a full body routine.

The problem with this argument is that after five sets of heavy bench press, your chest is already quite fatigued. You won't be able to bring the same intensity to subsequent chest exercises.

In a full body routine, you get the five intense sets of bench press, and then switch body parts and do something like heavy rows using your back (that's still fresh). In a split, you switch to incline bench, but can only do a percentage of your true capability, because your chest is already beat up from the flat bench press you started with.

The result is that you get significantly diminishing marginal returns. You extract far less value out of each subsequent exercise. This problem is side stepped with a full body routine, where you get the intense, bang-for-your-buck reps and then rest so you can get another dose of them a couple of days later, rather than having to wait a full week.

3. More Variety and More Intensity

The last reason the full body routine is king is a mental one.

Because you're only lifting weights three times per week, your enthusiasm will be higher each time you're at the gym. This will translate to more intensity. Also, because you're constantly switching between muscle groups, you're more likely to stay acutely focused to the exercise at hand.

 The benefits of using a full body routine, like the one found in this book, should be obvious to you at this point. The proof is in the pudding: all professional bodybuilders before the 60s or 70s used full body routines to build their impressive physiques. This includes guys like Arnold Schwarzenegger, Steve Reeves, Reg Park, and Leroy Colbert.

And while it's true that today's bodybuilders are bigger than they were back in the day, you must realize that the amount and variety of steroids used today is exponentially higher than ever before. This is the reason for the bigger physiques, not because some of them have switched to using split routines.

Chapter 17

What is the Optimal Way to Plan Your Meals?

A lot of discussion goes into the conversation of how many meals you should eat, when you should eat them, and how big they should be.

It's stupid.

In the end it doesn't matter.

Follow These Three "Rules" For Success

1. You should eat however many meals you want to.

2. You should eat them whenever you want to.

3. They should be as big or as small as you want them to be.

That's it. With the additional requirement that at the end of the day you should have eaten roughly your target number of total calories and sufficient protein, fiber, and vitamins.

Obsessing over these other factors is silly. I'll dispel the common myths below.

Don't Eat Late at Night

I frequently hear people asserting that eating at night is a bad idea, with the usual rational being that food consumed at late hours won't be used for energy, but instead automatically stored as body fat as you sleep.

Fortunately, overall energy balance is the only factor that leads to an increase in weight, and therefore body fat.

An example to illustrate this concept is as follows. Imagine that you wake up at 8 AM and eat a small breakfast of 500 calories. After a busy day at work you return home, without having eaten anything since breakfast. Throughout the day your body expended 3000 calories worth of energy. Hungry, you consume a massive 1500 calorie meal at 10PM, just before falling asleep.

The result? You consumed 2000 calories while expending 3000, yielding a deficit of 1000 calories. Yes, that means you lost weight, despite your large bedtime meal.

Eat This Before Your Workout

Contrary to common belief, eating a small meal before training is not necessary.

A recent study even found that fasted training can lead to a higher rate of protein synthesis after a workout (18).

That being said, many people report higher energy levels after consuming a small meal. Personally, I prefer lifting weights after waking up, but before eating anything.

Find out what works for you, and then do it. Man up and stop relying on other people's advice.

Eat This After Your Workout

Post workout nutrition is nearly universally hailed as the most important time to eat in the world of bodybuilding.

Many resources refer to a special window of 30 minutes to an hour after lifting weights when your body will magically turn everything you eat into muscle.

While a period of time does exist when rates of protein synthesis are raised after a workout, it turns out this window is better measured in hours or days, not minutes (4). This means you don't need to be sipping on a protein shake during your workout, or immediately after finishing your last repetition... unless you want to look like a fool.

In regards to what you should eat after a workout, recent studies show carbohydrate rich foods, along with at least a small amount of amino acids (protein) to be preferable (19). But even the data in this study suggests only marginal benefits.

I'll repeat the three rules to meal timing and planning one more time:

1. You should eat however many meals you want to.

2. You should eat them whenever you want to.

3. They should be as big or as small as you want them to be.

Just hit your target calories and get sufficient protein, fiber, and vitamins – end of discussion.

Chapter 18

What is the Optimal Protein/Carb/Fat Ratio?

After figuring out how many calories you need to eat, the next logical step is figuring out what combination of proteins, carbs, and fats will constitute these calories.

Proteins, carbs, and fats are collectively called the macro-nutrients. They are the three "types" of calories you can eat. All too often people get caught up thinking that fats are evil and carbs convert to fat or something stupid like that (hint: both of these notions are false).

I'll briefly cover what you need to know about each one.

1. Proteins

Your skin, muscles, organs, and glands are all composed of protein. It plays a major role in repairing cells and creating new ones. For this reason it's significant for growth and development – yes that means for your muscles, but also for key periods of your life in general (childhood, adolescence, etc.).

After proteins are digested, amino acids are what remain. They are required for breaking down food. There are a set of eight essential amino acids that the body needs, but cannot produce by itself (7).

A food containing all eight essential amino acids is called a complete protein. It's important to include some of these in your diet: eggs, milk, cheese, yogurt, meat, chicken, fish, beans, lentils, and peanuts (7). As you can see these cover just about all the commonly known protein sources. It should be easy to incorporate a few into your diet, if not already present.

Daily Requirement

For all of the above reasons, sufficient protein intake is important. General health recommendations dictate a minimum daily intake of 0.4 grams of protein per pound of bodyweight (0.88 grams per kg) (8).

Bodybuilding requirements tend to be far more demanding, with some sources recommending as much as 2 grams per pound of bodyweight (4.4 g/kg) daily. Don't do this. Your wallet will never forgive you.

As I mentioned earlier, current data suggests that strength athletes should consume roughly 0.8 grams per pound (1.75 g/kg) of bodyweight per day. I believe this number is sufficient to ensure maximum muscle gains while gaining weight and maximum muscle retention while losing weight.

Protein Synthesis & Muscle Growth

Understanding the exact process by which your muscles actually grow will shed more light on the importance of nutrition. Just as energy balance determines whether you gain or lose weight, a similar equation determines whether you lose or gain muscle.

The two processes of muscle protein breakdown and muscle protein synthesis are constantly in action. Muscle protein breakdown is the process through which proteins degrade into amino acids. Muscle protein synthesis is the process through which new proteins are created. Muscle growth only occurs when muscle protein synthesis exceeds muscle protein breakdown – a positive muscle protein balance must exist.

Someone in a state of positive protein muscle balance is referred to as anabolic, while someone in a negative balance is considered catabolic. While resistance training does improve muscle protein balance, it's impossible to be anabolic without consuming food (9).

2. Carbs

Unlike the other two macronutrients, carbohydrates are not required for any particular bodily functions. However, they are still useful because they provide a quality source of energy to the body (10).

The main distinction people make is between simple carbohydrates and complex carbohydrates (e.g. white vs. whole grain bread). This refers to the chemical composition of the food, and how fast it's digested.

Simple carbohydrates contain only one or two sugars and digest quickly while complex carbohydrates contain more and take longer to break down. As a result complex carbohydrates are usually attributed with providing longer lasting energy and are generally recommended.

However, this idea is given far too much importance because foods are not digested in isolation one-by-one, but rather as a part of an entire meal. Thus, if there are any fats, proteins, or other carbohydrates in your meal (and 99.9% of the time, there are) then this difference is entirely mitigated (11).

Fiber and the Micronutrients

Although not essential for bodily functions, some carbohydrate sources like fruits and vegetables contain micronutrients and fibers that are essential for a healthy body.

Micronutrients are nutrients that humans require to perform a variety of physiological functions, but are not produced naturally by our bodies. In general, this means vitamins and minerals.

Fiber is an indigestible carbohydrate. The two types of fiber are soluble fiber (dissolves in water) and insoluble fiber (does not break down when it passes through the digestive tract). Higher intakes of fiber are associated with regular bowel movements as well lower incidence of heart disease and some types of cancer. For this reason the recommended daily intake of fiber is 38 grams for men (12).

3. Fats

Fats do not make you fat. Only consuming more calories than you expend will cause weight gain.

In fact, fats are a vital part of every diet. Here are a couple reasons they must be eaten:

1. Fats are the only source of essential fatty acids, which are required by the body but cannot be produced by it naturally. In other words, they must be attained through food. The essential fatty acids play an important role in controlling inflammation, blood clotting, and brain development (13).

2. Fats help the body absorb and utilize vitamins A, D, E, and K and therefore are vital for healthy skin, hair, bones, and teeth (13).

It's also useful to be aware of the different types of fats:

1. Unsaturated Fats: These are preferable because they raise HDL levels (good cholesterol) and help prevent heart disease (14). Example food sources: olive oil, fish.

2. Saturated Fats: These are fine in moderation, but be aware – they raise LDL levels (bad cholesterol) (14). Example food sources: butter, cheese, ice cream, fatty meats.

3. Artificial Trans-Fats: These should be avoided as they both raise LDL levels and lower HDL levels (14). Example food sources: fried food, donuts, cookies, processed foods.

So what is the optimal ratio?

There isn't one. You should base your diet on your own personal needs, not an arbitrary ratio.

Follow these three steps:

1. Eat 0.8 grams of protein per pound of bodyweight (1.75 g/kg).

2. Eat a handful of healthy fats.

3. Eat fruits and vegetables every day.

...and fill the rest of your target calories however you want to.

Chapter 19

The Top 15 Cheap and Healthy Foods

Knowing how many calories and grams of protein you need is good, but finding the actual foods to construct your diet can be a pain in the ass.

In fact, most guys eat out all the time due to pure laziness (whether they want to improve their body or not). Being able to prepare a handful of quick and delicious meals will be a deciding factor in your success.

Not only is it a challenge to get an accurate estimate of how many calories you eat at a restaurant – eating out is also a lot more expensive. If you can cut down the number of meals you eat out to just one per day, your wallet and your body will both thank you.

Use the list below as starting point to kick off your journey as a master chef (of simplicity). All of the listed foods are nutritious, will help you reach your fitness goals, and are cheap. I've broken them down by whether they're primarily a source of proteins, carbs, or fats.

Protein Sources

1. Chicken breast

Why: It will get you the most grams of protein per dollar. It's also arguably the most versatile type of meat.

Sample Meals: Chicken breast with rice and vegetables, chopped up chicken breast stir fried with vegetables

2. Ground beef

Why: It's delicious.

Sample Meals: hamburgers, ground beef with rice and vegetables

Considerations: If you're in a weight loss phase go for the 90/10 (lower fat and lower calorie) or skip it altogether. If you're not, then go for the 80/20 or 85/15 because it's cheaper and the extra calories won't hurt you.

3. Ground turkey

Why: It's almost as delicious as ground beef. But it's good to switch things up, and it's a bit lower fat (if you're in a weight loss period, this is beneficial).

Sample Meals: The same as ground beef

4. Protein powder

Why: Convenience is the main factor here. If you're a busy person with little time to prepare meals it can come in handy. It's also arguably as cheap as chicken breasts depending on the brand you get.

Sample Meals: Protein shake (protein powder and milk), proats (see the next chapter)

Considerations: Generally going for what's cheapest is okay. There are too many options out there for me to cover each one but my two favorite brands are *Dymatize* and *Optimum Nutrition*.

5. Bacon

Why: It's the best breakfast food around.

Sample Meals: Bacon, eggs, and toast

Considerations: None.

Carb Sources

1. Rice

Why: It's one the cheapest carb sources you can buy, and it goes well with nearly any meal.

Sample Meals: Rice with vegetables and chicken, rice as a side to any piece of meat

Considerations: I prefer white rice because it tastes better and cooks in half the time of brown.

2. Quick oats

Why: It's very cheap, and you can combine it with nearly anything.

Sample Meals: Proats (see the next chapter)

Considerations: I only get the quick, one-minute variety. If you get regular or steel-cut be ready to put in more time to prepare them.

3. Sliced bread

Why: It's super cheap and can be used in a lot of meals.

Sample Meals: Any sandwich or hamburger, toast with butter.

4. Milk

Why: This could've been mentioned under protein sources, but it contains more carbs than protein. It also contains fats, and that's why it's awesome (it's a solid blend of proteins, carbs, *and* fats).

Sample Meals: Milk, chocolate milk, protein shake.

Considerations: If you're in a weight loss period, go for skim or 1%, but if you're not, go for 2% or whole.

5. Mixed frozen vegetables

Why: If you're like me then buying, preparing, and eating vegetables seems like a pain in the ass. Yes, I know they're important for my health, but they don't taste that good for all of the hassle required to prepare them.

Gentlemen, let me introduce you to frozen vegetables. They're cheap, you don't have to clean them, you just microwave or cook them in a frying pan with some olive oil, and they're often fresher than the fresh vegetables (because they're flash frozen on site).

Sample Meals: Eat them as a side to any meal, as part of a stir-fry, or omelet

Considerations: I usually get a few of the variety packs and a bag of broccoli florets.

6. Bananas

Why: It's the easiest to prepare (just peel it) and potentially the cheapest fruit you can buy.

7. Orange juice

Why: It's delicious and contains the same vitamins you'd find in an orange.

Considerations: Get the not-from-concentrate variety.

Fat Sources

1. Peanut butter

Why: It contains healthy fats and some protein. It's also incredibly cheap.

Sample Meals: Peanut butter and jelly sandwich, proats (see the next chapter), peanut butter and a banana

Considerations: Go for the natural variety. It's a little more expensive, but it cuts out the trans-fats and hydrogenated oils.

2. Buttery Spread

Why: It tastes better than butter and contains healthy fats like omega threes.

Sample Meals: Buttered toast, any meal that calls for butter during cooking

Considerations: I prefer the *Smart Balance* brand.

3. Eggs

Why: They're delicious and versatile. It could've been a protein source, but it's pretty high in fat if you eat the yolk (and you should – egg whites are for women).

Sample Meals: Bacon and eggs, vegetable omelet

Considerations: None.

Chapter 20

2 Cheap, Instant Muscle Building Meals

In the previous chapter I alluded to a couple of meals that I find borderline magical. Use these meals wisely and they'll make achieving your dietary goals far easier.

They're both delicious, can both be made in less than five minutes, and contain a good balance of fats, carbs, and proteins.

1. Proats

Proats is simply a combination of protein powder and oats. It generally involves protein powder, oats, milk, and a few mix-ins. The possibilities are nearly endless, but my favorite is definitely chocolate peanut butter proats – it's like a *Reese's* cup, but in oatmeal form.

Ingredients

- ½ to 1 cup quick oats

- ½ to 1 cup milk

- 1 scoop chocolate protein powder

- 2 tbsp. Peanut butter

Directions

1. Mix the milk and oats together in a bowl

2. Microwave (for one minute if you have quick oats, otherwise it will be longer)

3. Mix in the protein powder and peanut butter

Notes

The amount of milk you need to use will vary with the type of protein powder you have. Some powders soak up far more milk than others. The microwave time may vary, too – based on your preference.

Also depending on whether you're trying to lose or gain weight, you can adjust the ingredient amounts. Adding in more peanut butter, for example, will yield a lot of extra calories.

2. Peanut Butter and Banana Sandwich

This is another staple in my diet. Just like proats: it's healthy, satisfying, and scrumptious.

Ingredients

- 2 pieces sliced bread

- 2 tbsp. peanut butter

- 1 banana

Directions

1. Spread the peanut butter on one piece of bread

2. Slice up the banana and put the slices on the other piece of bread

3. Put the peanut butter covered slice on top of the banana covered slice and cut it in half

Notes

I'll repeat this: depending on whether you're trying to lose or gain weight, you can adjust the ingredient amounts. Adding in more peanut butter, for example, will yield a lot of extra calories.

Chapter 21

The Truth about Alcohol's Effects on Building Muscle and Cutting Fat

I included this chapter in the book because it's a question that guys ask me all the time. Here's the truth on how alcohols effects on your level of fitness.

Alcohol is effectively a fourth macronutrient, coming in at 7 calories per gram. Unfortunately, unlike the other 3 macronutrients (fats, carbohydrates, and proteins) your body isn't capable of efficiently deriving energy from it – hence the popular term *empty calories*.

This is misleading because some energy is, in fact, derived – just a smaller percentage. And this percentage decreases with subsequent drinks. This means that your body actually utilizes a substantial percentage of the calories consumed from the first couple of drinks for energy (23).

Furthermore, alcohol inhibits protein synthesis, and therefore can prevent optimal rates of muscle growth. However, it's important to note that the studies that confirm this notion have been performed on rats and alcoholics (24).

These facts have a couple of key implications.

1. In terms of weight or fat gain, energy balance is still king.

If you consume more calories than you expend (eat more than you burn) you will gain weight – regardless if alcohol was or was not included in said calories.

2. Heavy alcohol consumption will affect your progress in the gym.

Big surprise, right? Heavy drinking leads to less energy being derived from the beverages and suppresses the rate at which your body can synthesize muscle protein. Not to mention that your performance will suffer if you're dehydrated or work out with a hangover.

In conclusion, as long as you limit alcohol consumption to a moderate amount there will be little to no negative side effects in the quest to gain muscle, cut fat, and improve your physique.

And that wraps it all up. Set goals, stay focused, hit the gym hard, track your diet, and achieve the body of a Shredded Beast. Then enjoy the confidence and character development that come along with it.

Go beast it.

Can You Do Me a Favor?

Thank you for buying and reading my book. I'm confident that you're well on your way to a lean, muscular, and strong body if you follow what's written inside.

Before you go, I have a small favor to ask. Would you take a minute to write a brief blurb about this book on Amazon? Reviews are the best way for independent authors (like me) to get noticed and sell more books. I also read every review and use the feedback to write future revisions – and future books, even.

Please navigate to the book's page on Amazon (http://www.amazon.com/product-reviews/B00IM4GKQY) in order to leave a review.

Thank you.

My Other Books

If you enjoyed this book, I'm willing to bet you'd find my others pretty awesome, too.

1. *The Book of Alpha: 30 Rules I Followed to Radically Enhance My Confidence, Charisma, Productivity, Success, and Life* (#1 Bestseller for Men's Health)

2. *The Book of Bulking: Workouts, Groceries, and Meals for Building Muscle*

3. *The Simple Art of Bodybuilding: A Practical Guide to Training and Nutrition*

Scientific References

1. Laforgia, Joe, R. T. Withers, and C. J. Gore. "Effects of exercise intensity and duration on the excess post-exercise oxygen consumption." Journal of sports sciences 24.12 (2006): 1247-1264.

2. Layman, Donald K., et al. "Dietary protein and exercise have additive effects on body composition during weight loss in adult women." The Journal of nutrition 135.8 (2005): 1903-1910.

3. Lemon, P. W. "Protein and amino acid needs of the strength athlete." Int J Sport Nutr 1.2 (1991): 127-45.

4. MacDougall, J. Duncan, et al. "The time course for elevated muscle protein synthesis following heavy resistance exercise." Canadian journal of applied physiology 20.4 (1995): 480-486.

5. Sale, Digby G. "Neural adaptation to resistance training." Med Sci Sports Exerc 20.5 Suppl (1988): S135-45.

6. Faires VM. Thermodynamics. New York, NY: Macmillan, 1967.

7. Shils ME, Young VR. Modern Nutrition in Health and Disease, 7th ed. Philadelphia, PA: Lea & Febiger, 1988.

8. Manore MM. Exercise and the Institution of Medicine recommendations for nutrition. Current Sports Medicine Reports 2005;4(4):193-198.

9. Tipton KD, Wolfe RR. Exercise, protein metabolism, and muscle growth. International Journal of Sport Nutrition 2001;11(1):109-132.

10. Turcotte, Lorraine P., et al. "Impaired plasma FFA oxidation imposed by extreme CHO deficiency in contracting rat skeletal muscle." Journal of Applied Physiology 77.2 (1994): 517-525.

11. Järvi, A. E., et al. "The influence of food structure on postprandial metabolism in patients with non-insulin-dependent diabetes mellitus." The American journal of clinical nutrition 61.4 (1995): 837-842.

12. Ryan-Harshman, Milly, and Walid Aldoori. "New dietary reference intakes for macronutrients and fibre." Canadian family physician 52.2 (2006): 177-179.

13. Groff JL, Gropper SS, Hunt SM. Advanced Nutrition and Human Metabolism. St Paul, MN: West Publishing, 1995.

14. Simopoulos, Artemis P. "ω-3 fatty acids in the prevention management of cardiovascular disease." Canadian journal of physiology and pharmacology 75.3 (1997): 234-239.

15. Food and Nutrition Board. Dietary Reference Intakes for Energy, Carbohydrates, Fiber, Fat, Protein, and Amino Acids (Macronutrients). Washington, DC: National Academy of Sciences; 2002.

16. McDonald L. "What's my genetic muscular potential?" Body Recomposition. 2009.
<http://www.bodyrecomposition.com/muscle-gain/whats-my-genetic-muscular-potential.html>.

17. Karlsson J, Satlin B. "Lactase, ATP, and CP in working muscle during exhaustive exercise in man." Journal of Applied Physiology 1970;29(5):596-602.

18. Deldicque L, De Bock K, Maris M, et al. "Increased p70s6k phosphorylation during intake of a protein–carbohydrate drink following resistance exercise in the fasted state." European Journal Applied Physiology 2010;108(4):791-800.

19. Burke LM, Kiens B, Ivy JL. "Carbohydrates and fat for training and recovery." Journal of Sports Science 2004;22(1):15-30.

20. Guallar, Eliseo, et al. "Enough is enough: Stop wasting money on vitamin and mineral supplements." Annals of Internal Medicine 159.12 (2013): 850-851.

21. Rodacki, Cintia LN, et al. "Fish-oil supplementation enhances the effects of strength training in elderly women." The American journal of clinical nutrition95.2 (2012): 428-436.

22. Trivedi, Daksha P., Richard Doll, and Kay Tee Khaw. "Effect of four monthly oral vitamin D3 (cholecalciferol) supplementation on fractures and mortality in men and women living in the community: randomised double blind controlled trial." BMJ: British Medical Journal 326.7387 (2003): 469.

23. Lieber CS. "Perspectives: do alcohol calories count?" American Journal of Clinical Nutrition 1991;54(6):976-982.

24. Pacy, P. J., et al. "The effect of chronic alcohol ingestion on whole body and muscle protein synthesis—a stable isotope study." Alcohol and Alcoholism 1991;26(5-6):505-513.

25. Fagard RH. "Exercise is good for your blood pressure." Clinical and Experimental Pharmacology and Physiology 2006;33(9):853-856.